Springer Biographies

The books published in the Springer Biographies tell of the life and work of scholars, innovators, and pioneers in all fields of learning and throughout the ages. Prominent scientists and philosophers will feature, but so too will lesser known personalities whose significant contributions deserve greater recognition and whose remarkable life stories will stir and motivate readers. Authored by historians and other academic writers, the volumes describe and analyse the main achievements of their subjects in manner accessible to nonspecialists, interweaving these with salient aspects of the protagonists' personal lives. Autobiographies and memoirs also fall into the scope of the series.

Haralampos M. Moutsopoulos

Passion for Excellence

My Lifelong Journey into Medicine
and Public Service

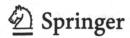 Springer

Haralampos M. Moutsopoulos (iD)
Academy of Athens
Section Sciences
Chair Medical Sciences-Immunology
Athens, Greece

ISSN 2365-0613   ISSN 2365-0621   (electronic)
Springer Biographies
ISBN 978-3-031-14130-0   ISBN 978-3-031-14128-7   (eBook)
https://doi.org/10.1007/978-3-031-14128-7

This Springer imprint is published by the registered company Springer Nature Switzerland AG
The registered company address is: Gewerbestrasse 11, 6330 Cham, Switzerland

There's nothin' you can do
that can't be done.
From the song "All you need is Love"
By The Beatles

Preface

I was born in the town of Ioannina in northwestern Greece, during World War II. I grew up during the Greek Civil War, and came of age during the prosperous years of reconstruction in the late 1950s and early 1960s, by which time I knew for certain that I wanted to practice medicine for the rest of my life. What follows is the story of my long medical career, and a chronicle of the many hurdles I encountered in my impassioned pursuit of knowledge and excellence.

This book was primarily written to honor all those who inspired me on this journey: my parents and my doctors, who first ignited my love for medicine; my teachers, who gave me, through their skill and example, the stimuli and the ability to acquire and produce medical knowledge; and finally, my associates, with whom I created two medical departments in Greece, offering excellent training to young doctors and producing new and innovative knowledge on autoimmune rheumatic diseases.

I have a faint hope that reading about the successes and failures documented in this book may be of interest to some people and helpful to others.

My higher purpose has always been to inspire young students and physicians to achieve excellence in medical knowledge, and also to provide an opportunity to those who are able and eager to produce new and novel medical data while instilling in them a sense of responsibility and a code of medical ethics.

This book has not omitted accounts of bitter experiences, unmanageable events, and trying situations. These were included because I do not adhere to the well-known adage that "one should not air one's dirty laundry in public." I believe that misconduct, if exposed, offers us collectively the chance to improve. I am not so much acting as a whistleblower but as an honest reporter. I am recording events, facts, and behavior as faithfully as possible, in the hope that my descriptions will expose what is wrong and will contribute to correcting it. I have never regretted anything I did. I was a demanding and exacting professor. I have often been called "domineering," "overzealous," "opinionated," and even "eccentric." I wear these characterizations as badges of honor. When the system is rotten, refraining from collusion is what is ethically required. When irrationality prevails, to be unreasonable is to be rational. When institutional behavior becomes ethically problematic, one has the duty to be eccentric or idiosyncratic. That is how I have tried to live my professional life. For this reason, it was not an easy life. But I would rather be remembered as an outspoken critic, who made life difficult for some, than as a tame sheep who followed the crowd.

I have always been driven by the Cretan novelist Nikos Kazantzakis' motto: "Embrace responsibility. Say: It is my duty, and mine alone, to save the earth. If it is not saved, then I alone am to blame." Well, I do not know about the earth in its entirety, but I did try to point my finger a little closer to home. I must also say that the frequent difficulties I encountered were counterbalanced by a good many moments of happiness, due first and foremost to the satisfaction of treating patients with autoimmune rheumatic disorders; due also to the joy of producing new medical knowledge and the pleasure of seeing our research work recognized by the international scientific community; and finally the delight of seeing my students progress to high academic positions both in Greece and abroad.

Athens, Greece   Haralampos M. Moutsopoulos

Acknowledgments

Special thanks are due to the following friends and colleagues for their constructive suggestions on the manuscript: my life companion, Fotini N. Skopouli, Nicolaos E. Madias, Spyros Retsas, Stuart S. Kassan, Gail Kassan, Clio P. Mavragani, Anthony Barnett, Richard Engler, and Alison Andritsopoulos.

I owe my gratitude also to Maria Tsirtsi for the meticulous editing of the manuscript as well as for her corrections in galley proofs.

Contents

About the Author

Professor Haralampos M. Moutsopoulos was born and raised in Ioannina, Greece. He received his M.D. and Ph.D. degrees from the National University of Athens and was trained in Internal Medicine at Georgetown University in Washington, D.C., and in Rheumatology/Immunology at the University of California, San Francisco. He worked as a scientist at the National Institutes of Health (NIH) and as Clinical Associate Professor of Medicine at Georgetown University Medical School, before returning to Greece as professor and Chairman at the University of Ioannina and then at the University of Athens Medical School. His research is focused on the understanding of the pathogenesis and the clinical expressions of autoimmune rheumatic diseases (ARD). Sjögren's syndrome is the prototype ARD disorder which he studies. His peer-reviewed scientific publications exceed 580 and are highly cited by his peers (citations >50000; h factor 115). He delivered several lectures in Rheumatology Immunology meetings and medical institutions in Europe, the USA, Mexico, Argentina, Brazil, Chile, Australia, Israel, Jordan, Japan, the USSR, and China, and worked as a visiting professor at Brest Medical School (France), at the University of California at Davis, at the University of Texas, in San Antonio, and at the Hospital of Special Surgery of Cornel Medical School, in NY. Springer has published two books that he edited and authored on Sjögren's syndrome, and recently a book entitled "Rheumatology in Questions" and its second revised edition "Immunology-Rheumatology in Questions". He is a recipient of significant national and international awards. More specifically, he received an award from the Hellenic Society of **Immunology** (2001) and he also received the **"Xanthopoulos-Pneumatikos"** Prize for his **excellence in university teaching** (2005), the **Bodosaki Excellence Award** (2010), granted by an international panel of experts, the **"Alessandro Robecchi"** Prize for Rheumatology research by EULAR (1987), the **European-Australian** Award for Medical Research (1993), **"Distinguished Scholar Clinician Award"** by ACR (2006), the **"Charles Von Pirquet"** Award for distinction in Medicine and Immunology (2007) by the University of California, Davis, the Title of **Hippocratic Orator** by the Hellenic Medical Society, London, U.K. (2008), the Title of **Master by the American College of Rheumatology** (2009), and the **Meritorious Service Award** (2010) for his outstanding services to Rheumatology by the EURAR. In

2014, the **President of the Hellenic Republic** decorated him with the **"Medal of Honor"** for his contribution to higher education and novel achievements in research. Furthermore, he is an Honorary member of the British Society of Rheumatology, a Fellow of the American College of Physicians and the Royal College of Physicians, and a life member of the Academy of Athens holding the Chair of Medical Sciences-Immunology in Science Section.

Chapter 1
Coming of Age

I was born and raised in Ioannina, a lovely garden city with a long tradition in "weapons, coins, and letters." My mother was from the Lappas family, who were considered "notables" (Photo 1.1). They were among the best-known lumber merchants in Greece. My mother's genealogical tree dates back more than 300 years. Their mansion on the island of Lake Pamvotis in Ioannina, where we spent our summers, was built on a large tract of land on the edge of the lake. It was comprised of three houses: the first and the second were built at the beginning of the nineteenth century, and the third at the end of that century. Across from the main house loomed Mitsikeli, the mountain that overlooks Ioannina. The house had its own small harbor. In the place where the lake and the back wall of the harbor met, there was cold, crystal-clear, drinkable water flowing. In the summer, it was used as a reserve icebox for fruit. In the center of the large stone-paved yard stood a large, hundred-year-old plane tree that provided natural shade for gatherings in summer. In the old days, the house was always open. It hosted meetings of politicians, scientists, and important figures in the local economy. The pater familias was Diamantis Lappas, my great-grandfather's brother, a lyricist, poet, and worshiper of beautiful women. He stayed single in order to raise the children of his brother, who died early. He left us nine hand-written manuscripts, three hundred pages each, which my mother guarded like the most precious treasure. When I retired from my post as professor, I studied these manuscripts and used the material in them to publish three books: the first contains poems, the second inlcudes advice from a self-taught person on health and disease, and the third one presents a collection of poetry, prose, and popular sayings. He never published these works, because they were written for his own satisfaction.

During the German Occupation, the family mansion was requisitioned by the Germans. It became Gestapo headquarters. It was there that Kurt Waldheim first landed. He was the one who gave the order for the arrest of the Jews of our city. Or so it was passed down by word of mouth for many years to come. The Occupation forces left the mark of their crass, barbaric, and senseless behavior on our house, as can be seen in scenes painted on the ceilings by local artists. They carry wounds that

© The Author(s), under exclusive license to Springer Nature Switzerland AG 2022
H. M. Moutsopoulos, *Passion for Excellence*, Springer Biographies,
https://doi.org/10.1007/978-3-031-14128-7_1

Photo 1.1 Mother Niki and father Michalis on their wedding day

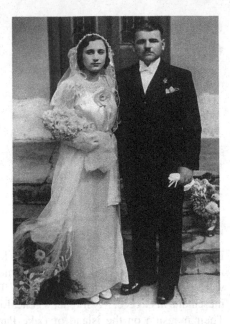

are still deep: eyes gouged from exotic multi-colored birds, and beautiful areas of Ioannina pierced by bullets are all that are still visible from their shooting matches.

Another part of our life on my mother's side of the family was taken up by the worship of God. The family gave the church three monastics: Friar Avakoum, Bishop Meletios, and Friar Grigorios. Each in his turn served as abbot in the monasteries of the Island of Ioannina.

My father's family was from Zagori. My grandfather was a merchant in Trieste. He had started another family there. His children, in Greece, were brought up by my grandmother Anna. Through sacrifices and hard work, they acquired an education that was unusual in those days.

My father, an honor student at the Agricultural School of Larissa, made use of a state scholarship to continue his studies for four years at the Agricultural School of Florence. When he returned, he was the only specialized arborist for plant disease and insects in Greece. In addition to his excellent technical education, he was also a student of poetry and of literature and would recite bits of literature to us by Krystallis, Papadiamantis, and Dante. He had an unusually strong personality and deep moral values. He was athletic, indifferent to worldly delights, and completely devoted to his work. His handwriting looked like a calligrapher's. He spent many days away from home touring various villages in Epirus. He adored agriculture. His trips to the villages were made so he could give advice to the villagers about how to improve their crops, take care of their trees and fight diseases (Photo 1.2). He behaved toward the farmers as if he was one of them. Without ever complaining and with great pleasure, he took on the chores of an agricultural technician. In his small suitcase, which he had picked up in Florence, he always carried a grafter, a clipper, and a magnifying

Photo 1.2 Author's father teaching olive growers how to control olive tree flies

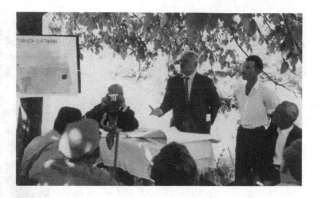

glass. He wrote two books: *The Apricot Tree*, in 1935 and *The Peach Tree*, in 1940. Both books were published by the Hellenic Agricultural Society. His books received highly favorable comments from the academic agricultural community. Experts in the field say that the data contained in these books is still applicable to good arboriculture practice even today.

Family was the other important part of his life. He gladly made great sacrifices to earn extra money for his children. On his trips, his expenses were minimal. Food was sparse: bread, olives and cheese, tomatoes, and occasionally a piece of smoked herring. Whatever the farmers gave him, a few apples, pears, and other fruit, he brought back to his family. When his trips were over, if he couldn't find any means of transportation, he would return home on foot, walking for hours. On Sundays, he was always the first person in church, when the first bell rang. He wanted to be next to the cantor, and sing along under his breath. He did not have a particularly good voice.

Our mother Niki, always well attired, paid great attention to the appearance of the other members of the family. Clever, and very well educated, she was both in love with and proud of her husband. She was very social, but she would not have visitors to the house unless she was properly dressed and her hair was done. She carried this refined background of hers throughout her life and cared deeply about maintaining her family's good standing in the community. Our father was very dependent on her care. Although in appearance she was subordinate to our father, she was in charge of all of the family decisions. She was the strict teacher of her children. She would draw our attention to danger, forbid things to us, and take precautions. That tender, loving, easily moved, caring mother would turn into an austere chastiser whenever we did something beyond the bounds she had set. She would raise her hand often. A slap from her was a painful and noisy punishment. In contrast, our father never scolded us. When our mother was young, she had wanted to study medicine. But her family circumstances did not permit it. So she channeled all her passion into her household, into the upbringing and education of her children.

Every night before we went to bed, our homework had to be checked by our mother. She knew Greek literature inside out. Her knowledge of the sciences was not far behind. She was a graduate of the Zosimaia High School, the most selective

Photo 1.3 Author's
siblings. From left to right:
author, Diamantis, and
Nikos. On the back Anna
embracing her brothers

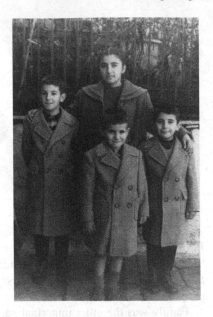

high school in the region of Epirus, which required entrance exams. Always first in
her class, she spoke French and played the mandolin. Her morals were exemplary.
She was well respected by her classmates. She would check all our notebooks, and
ask us questions to see how well prepared we were. If she found any mistakes, she
wouldn't let us go to bed until we had corrected them. Her dream was for us to
always be first, the ones who would stand out in life and in society. She excelled at
cooking, sewing, and embroidery. Every season when the trees in our garden bore
fruit—plums, apricots, cherries—or when the market was filled with tangerines and
eggplant, our house would be turned into a sweet-maker's workshop. The shelves in
our buffet would fill up with a variety of sweets in glass jars, so we would be ready to
offer homemade sweets to any visitors who might come to our house. My mother's
talents did not go unnoticed by Ioannina society. She served as a cooking, baking,
and handiwork advisor to the ladies of her generation around the city.

There were four of us siblings (Photo 1.3). I was the second-born and made my
appearance seven years after my sister Anna, who, brought up to be a good daughter,
also acted as mother. An excellent student and violinist, Anna studied at the Zosimaia
Pedagogical Academy. In addition to getting educated, she was being prepared for
the roles of wife and mother. Nikos, unusually clever, always first in his class but
also first in crazy pranks, and the ringleader of his classmates, was studying to be
an engineer. Diamantis also got into the pedagogical academy, but he chose not to
pursue his studies. From an early age, he had many health problems. With the help
of our father, he was appointed an employee in a local manufacturing firm. He was
very well liked by his classmates, his co-workers, and his friends. He was sensitive,
and although he was an introvert, he was also quite social.

As for me, I was a happy and clever child, well behaved, fond of hugs and kisses—a child that everyone, not only the family but also our friends, found to be delightful. Memories from those years keep coming back to me. How can one forget the bear-keeper with his tambourine and the bear, chained to his cart, wandering the streets of the city? The bear, aside from entertaining us, acted as a physiotherapist. Many people, particularly women, would come and lie on their stomachs in the street and enjoy the bear's healing footsteps on their backs. Those poor people believed that the applied pressure of bear's foot would cure their back pain. And the fisherman from the island, with fresh, pan-broiled, oregano-spiced crayfish, going around with his goods to the coffee shops in the central square, and the salep-peddler with his cart, roaming the streets of Ioannina.

This was back in the years of the Civil War when there was so much killing on both sides. It was forbidden to circulate after 6 p.m. The streets and alleys of the city looked ravaged. It looked like a dead city. Here and there you could see a few people in the street like ghosts.

One winter afternoon, our parents and Anna went to attend some social event. We younger children stayed at home with the housekeeper. When they came back just before sunset, they found us in an awful state. Nikos had managed to stuff a metal button he had cut from his shirt up his nostril. In a jiffy, our father picked him up and, despite the curfew, took him to the nearest ear, nose, and throat specialist. The doctor tried his hardest to remove the button from Nikos nostril but did not succeed. Our father, without wasting another moment, took Nikos to the best-known surgeon in Ioannina, Dr. Danos, who dislodged the button with a single motion. He simply used a magnet and pulled it out. After this successful operation, he turned to my father and asked him, with feigned innocence, who had tried to remove the button before him. "Well, it was So-and-So," replied my father. "So, Michalis, did you forget that Danos is here in Ioannina? This mistake will now cost you one gold sovereign." He was terribly money-minded, that ungodly soul. He and the general practitioner, Dr. Defteraios, had brought the first X-ray machine to Ioannina. One night, at the central coffee shop of Ioannina, they asked him what he saw with that machine. "What I see," he answered, "are fifty-drachma bills. What my colleague sees, God only knows."

I still cannot forget the agony and fear that gripped us back then, waiting for my father to return, when he was called to Security Police Headquarters. He was often summoned there for questioning and explanations. Our house was under surveillance. They wanted to know who came and went. Most of my father's relatives, and my father himself, you see, had a record. A file had been created by the nationalists when the civil war ended. There were many accusations in it, both from the period of the Occupation and the Civil War period immediately following. Buying a left-leaning Athens daily newspaper was quite an adventure. Every day we went to a different kiosk in a different neighborhood of Ioannina. We never carried the newspaper in plain sight. We carried it home, well hidden under our clothing, like a treasure.

Our toys were for the most part made by our parents or by older friends, from whatever material was available. The ball bearings from various engines were precious and hard to find. You couldn't make a skateboard without them. Two-pronged branches from trees were used to make slingshots, necessary weapons for children of our age.

Used inner tubes were made into lifejackets or boats to be played with in the waters of Lake Pamvotis. Our allowances were used to purchase marbles of different sizes and colors. We had quite a large collection. Whenever we had lamb for a meal, we would fight over who would get the talus bone. After cleaning and bleaching it in limewater, it was ready to be used as a toy. The talus was thrown, and the person who guessed which side would be up was the winner.

We were among the luckier kids in the neighborhood. We had musical instruments in our house: our sister's violin and our mother's mandolin. The orchestra was completed with the lids of pots and pans and a makeshift tambourine. The "music hall" for this orchestra was a very large built-in closet. We called it the "chamber." It was there that we created our symphonic compositions. It was the space that we used for many years as a retreat. It was our hiding place. The performances of our compositions took place when our parents and our sister were out at social gatherings. We also had a *Bianchi* athlete's bicycle, a late 1920s model. Our father had purchased it during his studies in Florence. We took turns riding it, and kept a list of who used it last.

We usually spent our summer vacations on the Island of Ioannina. It was there that we first learned to swim. Fishing in the lake and playing on the island's small hill were what normally kept us busy. Only rarely, one summer maybe two, did we spend our vacation at the seaside town of Ipsos, in Corfu.

Our main residence, a private nineteenth-century house, in the center of Ioannina, which was part of my mother's dowry, had large, spacious rooms and huge windows that allowed a lot of sun to shine in. We spent most of the year in that house.

The sitting room and the formal dining room were out of bounds for us. They were "museum" rooms that were opened only on name days and during the Christmas holidays, or for certain special guests, who would appear every now and then.

The sitting room was filled with furniture. The buffet with the glass showcase was always locked. This was done to keep the jarred candied fruits away from the children. Those sweets were only for visitors. On the two large walls of this room, in the most prominent place, were several large-framed photographs of our grandmothers, my father's mother, and my mother's mother. In the dining room, which was only used for very formal dinners, hung the photographs of our grandfathers. The large sitting room was where the family gathered for meals. But it was also my father's office and my mother's workshop. It had a Singer sewing machine in one corner, and in the middle a fireplace that was never lit. Majestically deployed along the walls were built-in wooden couches. Next to them were the bookcases. Like all the furniture in the house, they were made in our grandfather's workshop out of thick walnut wood. Hand-embroidered short curtains decorated the glass panes of these bookcases, to protect the leather spines of the books from the sun's rays. The bookcases contained a wealth of materials: encyclopedias, collections of poetry, short stories, novels, and of course all sorts of books on agriculture in French, Italian, and Greek. In the other corner was a table that my father used for reading and writing.

The eastern corner of the room housed the iconostasis. Thanks to my mother's care, a candle burned day and night in front of icons of the Virgin Mary's sweet visage and of otherworldly, ascetic forms of saints, whose names corresponded to those of members of our family.

The room we used for studying was on the first floor and had plenty of sun. Next to this room were the living quarters of our housekeeper. Also on the first floor were three large family bedrooms: one for Anna, one for the boys and one for my parents. My parents' bedroom was next to ours. We were separated only by a thick, multi-leaf folding door. Many evenings, when I couldn't sleep, I was privy to their erotic couplings. I was never frightened by their groans and the squeaking sounds of their creaky, walnut-wood bed. Those experiences made me aware of the sexual act. It was an immediate, unexpected education.

Grandpa Nikolaos Moutsopoulos' bedroom was on the same floor, but off-limits to us. It was always ready to welcome him on his rare visits to us from Trieste. I don't remember much about him. The only strong memories that have stayed with me are the lively arguments he had with my father. There was a toilet on every floor of the house. On the ground floor, there was a second toilet for guests. We didn't acquire a proper bathroom until the 1960s.

Every Saturday afternoon was devoted to bodily cleanliness for the whole family. It began with bathing the children and ended with the housekeeper bathing herself. A large quantity of water was heated in a cauldron in the washhouse. In the 1940s and 1950s, the bathtub was made out of enamel, and it was movable.

Winters in Ioannina were very cold. Often the scuppers were adorned with icicles. It was not an unusual sight for the city to be covered in snow and the lake frozen over. Before we acquired central heating in 1960, we kept warm using wood-burning stoves and coal-burning pans. The heat they emitted gave off a feeling of coziness.

We also had the good fortune of having a large garden, spread out over four levels between two parallel roads. The yard in the back of the house was paved. It was adorned with pots with a variety of flowers. On the second level, all kinds of vegetables were grown. On the right of this level, a marble well stood proudly. It was always filled with water, ready to quench the thirst of plants, flowers, and trees. On the left, was the washhouse, a separate, stone building. Half of it was a storage area for firewood and our father's agricultural equipment, and the other half was used as a working space for the women of the house. It had a large sink and a section like a fireplace for boiling vast quantities of water in huge cauldrons. That's where they did the laundry, before we acquired a washing machine in the 1960s. It was also the place where wool was dyed to be woven into various items for the family. And finally, it served as the slaughterhouse for hens, roosters, goats, and sheep. Every Christmas and Easter, a lamb would arrive from grandfather's farm in Petra, Preveza. Our father performed the sacrificial skinning and thorough cleansing of the innards of the lamb. Our mother used their tiny feet and stomach to make a delicious soup called *patsá*, while the innards were braided and roasted with the intestines and with vegetables for the Good Saturday (Resurrection) feast. In the third section of the garden stood our chicken coop. It provided us with organic eggs and plenty of meat, from the hens in the winter, and in the summer from the roosters.

The fourth level was the orchard. It looked like a forest to us. Filled with fruit-bearing trees, this garden was my father's pride and joy. He tended to the trees with great care. He caressed them, talked to them, and took care of all their needs. He believed they communicated with him. Our garden provided us with plenty of fruit, vegetables, and flowers of all kinds. They were all our own produce. Our father always taught us that what grows in the earth must only be eaten when in season. He did not believe in defiling nature. We would climb the trees like Tarzan. The foliage of the fig tree and the other thick-branched, fruit-bearing trees made the tree orchard an ideal hiding place. We would split up into teams and play cowboys and Indians. We were very careful not to step on and destroy the flower garden and the vegetable garden.

Many years have passed since then, but I am still very attached to that house. It was and remains important, not because it had simple, beautiful furniture and a nourishing garden, but because it was the center of my social upbringing. It was there that I learned to deal maturely with difficulties, and to speak openly without fear. It was there that I internalized the meanings of love, truth, and honesty. Every time I return there, it calms me and restores me spiritually. It is our hope to keep it as it is. We do not want to replace it with an impersonal apartment building. After my parents' death, I renovated the house. The furniture, dating back to the middle of the nineteenth century, was all polished. A large part of my art collection was hung on the walls of the house, which is now like a real museum. I want it to live on, unchanged forever, to retain both the happy and the unpleasant memories. I would love for my children and their descendants to stay there, when they visit Ioannina.

The schools were also gravely damaged by the Italian and German bombardments. The nursery school was housed in the Monastery of St. Catherine, about 100 yards to the left of our house. The primary school was located in a corrugated metal shed, a gift from the Marshall Plan. In the winter, every student had to cart firewood with him, the amount depending on his strength, for the wood-burning stove. All our teachers took great interest in our intellectual development. They were the epitome of devoted spiritual counselors, with no interest in enriching themselves or promoting themselves socially. I was teacher's pet to my favorite teacher, Xenophon Tzavellas. He treated me with the care of a father. He had no children. His students filled this void.

In the last classes of primary school, I began extracurricular activities, such as English lessons, studying Byzantine music, and sports. Our English teacher was named Kalliopitsa Hatzi, the only daughter of a prominent family. She lived with her housekeeper and many cats. Her house was a few doors away from ours. She was permissive, not at all hard-handed. Her class hour was spent playing games. Her cats were our favorite playthings. We spent more time playing with them than learning English. We cloaked our indifference to foreign languages in a patriotic mind-set. We did not want to learn the language of the foreigners who had occupied Cyprus. This was our understanding of the world in our patriotic childhood minds back then.

The teacher of Byzantine music also taught religion to us. His unpleasant personality made me finish very quickly with that not-so-interesting educational experience.

Sports—I was a sprinter running the 100- and 200-yard dashes—took care of my excess energy. I trained in the afternoon, practically every day, at the Ioannina

Stadium, which, luckily for me, was quite near my house. I was a fast runner and became a valuable member of our school athletic team. But my involvement in sports ended ingloriously. In the spring of 1957, after an intense workout, sweating profusely, I sat down to rest on the steps of the yard. I awoke the next day unable to walk. This weakness spread further, until it confined me to bed. My feet felt like two sacks of cement. I couldn't lift them. My doctors, Giorgos Fotiadis, a neurologist, Nikos Skopoulis, a pediatrician, and Giorgos Melanidis, an internist, examined me individually and in consultation. I understood that they could not figure out what was wrong with me. Their compassion for me was moving, but their treatment was painful, consisting of intramuscular injections with large doses of penicillin, and catastrophic for my appearance, because of the large doses of cortisone. All this kept me in bed for over a month. Many years later, I was able to diagnose myself: acute, post-infection polyneuropathy, or Guillain-Barré syndrome. Fortunately, the paralysis did not continue up past my lower limbs. The treatment I was given then, as we know today, many years later, is ineffective for that particular illness and could quite possibly worsen the condition. Though we know today that the syndrome in question was an autoimmune polyneuritis, back then even autoimmune disorders were unknown. After my recovery, the doctors' orders were clear: avoid all exercise. So that was the inglorious end to my possibly glorious athletic career.

Starting in primary school, we children and others from the neighborhood served as altar boys. We helped out at Mass. After a fight, the strongest boy would get to carry the cross and the others the cherubim. Confession and Communion were strictly scheduled by our mother. These activities came quickly to an end, however. Our confessor was very strict, and it was difficult for us adolescents to follow his orders.

In 1956, after passing the entrance exams, I was enrolled at the highly competitive Zosimaia High School, part of a nation-wide system of what are known as prototype public schools to prepare promising students for university. I was now a student of a well-known educational institution. In the second year of junior high school, our school moved from an old, dilapidated building to the newly built Zosimaia School, a few meters from our house. It had large, sun-filled classrooms, modern laboratories, and a courtyard large enough for sports. Our interactions with the teachers varied. Many were excellent teachers in their fields, but difficult individuals. I won't forget the maths teacher. He was tall, well dressed, a loner, sullen, strict, and narcissistic. Without reservations, he stressed to us that he was an expert and that the grade of "excellent" was for him only. The highest grade he gave on oral exams was fourteen out of twenty. But we acquired a solid foundation in mathematics from that teacher.

Other teachers were kind and sympathetic when it came to children's problems. Our French teacher, Arsenis Gerontikos, in spite of an imperious expression and a penetrating stare, was one of them. Our French class was an hour of philosophy, sociology, and literature. I don't believe there is a single student who took a class with him and didn't adore him. Equally memorable is the stern, self-centered, but gentle, personality of our Ancient and Modern Greek teacher, Sotiris Nikolos. He knew everything there was to know about Greek literature and history. His enthusiasm was contagious. We would hang on his every word. He was earnest and passionate, when

Photo 1.4 Author (left)
with grandfather and brother
Nikos (right), and cousin
Kostas (front)

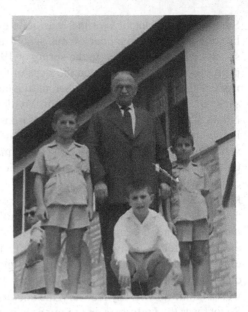

he spoke to us. He was so excited by teaching that when he spoke, he spewed saliva
all over us. Fortunately, very few teachers discriminated against students based on
the political leanings of their parents. A sad example of such behavior was the teacher
of religion. All the children of parents "under investigation" were stigmatized and
received very low grades in oral exams. I don't think there were any students who
liked or respected him.

My maternal grandfather Lousias, a nickname for Haralampos, was my encyclo-
pedia. We took great pleasure in our outings with him (Photo 1.4). He described
things so beautifully and vividly that not even the best storyteller could compete
with him.

When I was with him, I had the opportunity to ask him thousands of questions. I
had many things on my mind. I'm afraid that, without wanting to, I became tiresome. I
wore him out. But I could see that, in spite of his tiredness, he enjoyed our discussions.
He provided answers to various social, economic, political, and existential questions
of mine. He was self-taught, with a wide range of economic, social, and historical
knowledge. He was obliged, after the premature death of his father, to take over the
business. He had the reputation of being a reasonable man and an astute analyst of the
economic events of his times. His fellow businessmen considered him trustworthy
and used him as an advisor and a banker. He wanted me to follow in his footsteps
and take over the business. But all of his efforts failed.

Grandma Harikleia adored us. She was our confidante when it came to our love
lives. She grew up in Ikonio, in Asia Minor. Because of this, her social mores were
far more liberal than those of the other ladies in Ioannina. I was the most loved of all
four siblings by my grandparents. I often spent weekends with them at their house

in the Castle, in the old city of Ioannina. It was there that my grandmother taught me to drink coffee.

My happy educational moments with my grandfather ended abruptly. I was in my second year of junior high school, when one day my grandmother notified that grandpa was having severe chest pain. By the time we arrived at his house, the doctor had diagnosed acute myocardial infarction. The only treatments back then were bed rest, painkillers and oxygen. He did not suffer a lot. On the second day of his illness he left us forever. I was by his side when he died.

It was a tradition in Lousias family for one of the grandsons to be in charge of running the monastery on the Island of Ioannina. He had to replace Master Grigorios, the theologian, who had studied at the Theology School of Chalkis, in Turkey, and the last monastic of the Ioannina monasteries from the family. The young man in question from the family had to have a penchant for religion and would study theology at the Theological School of Chalkis. But he would have to devote himself to God, forsake worldly pursuits and become a monk. All of the boys in the family declined this invitation.

My first amorous awakenings were in the last classes of primary school. There was a beautiful girl there. She was taller than me. I thought she admired the fact that I was a good student. The most gratifying part of our relationship was when we walked home from school holding hands.

My adolescence began early in junior high school. I will never forget the woman who, several years later, would undertake my sexual education. She was dark-haired, with fiery eyes, incredible curves, saucy, and womanly. I have to admit that my experience with her had nothing at all in common with my first platonic love.

I had got it into my head from an early age that I would become a physician. It is possible that this wish of mine was due to my mother's unfulfilled desire to study medicine, or perhaps my childhood illnesses played some role, or the example of the professionalism and empathy with which my doctors treated me. Although all of us boys were good students, we had a particular penchant for science, and especially mathematics. My main interest was in the human body, in understanding its biology. I pored through many books on biology outside of school. My interest in man and in death led me on many occasions to attend funerals in the church of my parish, the Archimandrio.

My last two years of high school were completed in Athens, at the First Prototype Boys' High School, in Plaka. Nikos, a year younger than me, was also enrolled there. We left Ioannina, mainly because we felt that in Athens we would be even better prepared for the university entrance examinations.

Our parents found a family, at 1 Plapouta Street in Exarchia, who were happy to have us as boarders. The building was old and had no elevator or central heating. After all the space we had in Ioannina, we now found ourselves in a tiny room that was barely big enough for us. The only pieces of furniture there were two beds and a table with two chairs. No one knew anyone else in that apartment building. No one knew whose birthday was or who had died. The walls kept them strictly separated. Without realizing it, I began to compare it to my previous surroundings. In Ioannina, wherever we went, for a walk, to the shops, to the main square, to the island, we knew everyone, friends, or relatives. Athens was a big change for us, which distressed and disappointed us. Our daily treks, morning and midday, from Exarchia to Plaka and back, our classes at school and our intensive studying after school for the university entrance exams left little time for the pleasures of old. We had no time to feel miserable either. Our supervisors and tender protectors that year were my grandmother's sister Meni and her husband, Christos Yeroyiannis, the high school principal. They lived far from us, in Dafni. Every Sunday, we had a good meal at their house, we talked over our problems and felt, for at least a few hours, the warmth of family. Great Aunt Meni had the comportment of an aristocrat. Great Uncle Christos, on the outside quite strict, was in fact a softie. The other member of the family was their son, Pavlos. An only child, he was a student at the Athens Polytechnic School.

I took entrance exams for the university medical schools in Athens and Thessaloniki, as well as for the Dental School of Athens University. Back then, there were no standardized pan-Hellenic entrance exams for higher educational institutions. I was accepted at all of them, among the top-ten students for the medical school in Thessaloniki and the dental school in Athens, but I was much lower on the list for the medical school of Athens. My grades on the essays pulled me down. But my goal and my dreams had been realized. I was now a medical student.

Chapter 2
Student Years

My admission to university brought its rewards. My parents decided to take us out of the prison of the tiny room in the apartment building on Plapouta Street. After brief visits to various apartments for rent, the right apartment was found. It was on the top floor of the "blue" apartment building in Exarchia Square. It was the best-known building in that area back then. It was large and imposing. It was surrounded by two-storey houses with balconies and gardens. Our apartment was bordered by a large terrace. From that terrace we could see all the famous sights of Athens—the Acropolis, Philopappos Hill and Lycabettus Hill. We could see all the way to the sea. Our apartment had yet another advantage. We could clandestinely watch the movies being shown in the outdoor movie theater across from us. The apartment was comfortable; we each had our own room.

Our mother, whose main interest in life was her children, decided to leave the city she loved and her house on Valaoritou Street in Ioannina, and come with us to Athens. We accepted this with mixed feelings. On the one hand happily, because we would always have impeccably clean clothes, home-cooked meals, and a clean house, but, on the other hand, our freedom would be curtailed by her vigilant surveillance. We had no choice. We came to terms with it, reasoning that there would be benefits from her presence. Our father stayed behind in Ioannina by himself. He had three more years to complete, before he retired.

My first year of studies at the Athens University Medical School went by quickly, a fun-filled, carefree year. My courses—chemistry (organic and inorganic), physics, and biology—were taught in a completely indifferent way; just a repeat of the material from high school. None of it had anything to do with medicine, and none of it was new. There was no connection between basic and applied science. Restless by nature, I kept looking for something interesting to keep me busy. My experience from home and the influence of my friends and fellow students led me to become involved in student politics. The Organization of Students from Epirus was made up of two factions: the Democrats and the Right. My heart was with the Democrats. I joined the organization. We met two or three times a week, in the afternoon, at the offices of the Democratic students on Solonos Street. We thought we could change the world.

© The Author(s), under exclusive license to Springer Nature Switzerland AG 2022   13
H. M. Moutsopoulos, *Passion for Excellence*, Springer Biographies,
https://doi.org/10.1007/978-3-031-14128-7_2

We discussed and recorded student problems, such as housing, meals, textbooks, funding for education, and other issues. We wrote up proposals and we prepared articles for the press. In the spring of 1963, during the elections for the appointment of the new administrative council of the organization, our opposing views were not confined to words, but we actually came to blows. Chairs were broken, clothing was torn, faces were bloodied, and bodies bruised. This brought to mind my parents' admonitions. Mostly my mother's, because she was frail and fearful by nature. "Let's not have the problems and rushing around we had with your father"; "Don't get involved in politics." "Finish your studies and try through your work to be of service to society and your country." And so my participation in these meetings began tapering off, and by my second year of studies it had stopped altogether.

In June, I took my exams with a very little studying and reviewing, and I passed. Without the knowledge that the following year courses in medicine would begin, my experience during my first year might have been a negative factor in my subsequent development as a man of medical science.

When the exams were over, I returned to the family home. Eight hours on a pre-war bus that only barely fit on the road from Athens to Ioannina. After a few days of enjoying the comforts of our home on the island, the summer program began: swimming at Limnopoula, a beach in Ioannina, or in the island; outings in the evening on the promenade or to the "bride's fair" in the town square; and perhaps once a week we would go to the movies. Reading things unrelated to medicine was of no particular interest to me, so I did very little of it. I found life there boring. I needed to find something to do that was connected to medicine. I quickly came to a decision. I thought it might be a good idea to go and work at the Hatzicostas Hospital. I wanted to be exposed to the beauty of my profession.

The hospital was a pleasant two-story classical revival building in a lovely flower garden. The arrangement of the flowers created the impression of abstract art with lively colors. The garden had been designed, constructed, and kept in excellent condition by the ongoing care of my father. The classical revival building was connected by a skywalk to a modern structure that looked like a matchbox. It had three departments: internal medicine, surgery, and pediatrics, and two diagnostic laboratories: clinical pathology and radiology, and outpatient clinics.

Without wasting any time, I decided to put my thoughts into action. I met with all the doctors, in all fields. I knew them all from my childhood years. They were most welcoming, but did not hide their dismay."Why do you want to work here so soon? You'll get tired of spending your life working with illness and sick people." I was not influenced by their comments. My desire and my adherence to my goals were so great that their advice went in one ear and out the other. After I visited all the departments, I found the area that inspired me, consisting of two or three rooms on the ground floor of the hospital: it was the clinical pathology laboratory.

The laboratory was dominated by the tall, upright, imposing figure of Dr. Achilleas Maroufof (Photo 2.1), a man of few words. He was assisted by a nurse, Georgia, and two lab assistants, Eftychia and Olga. Politely, discreetly and patiently, I tried to figure out what they did. Eftychia showed me around the lab. She showed me all the laboratories: hematology, biochemistry, and microbiology. She explained how

Photo 2.1 Dr. Achilleas
Maroufof

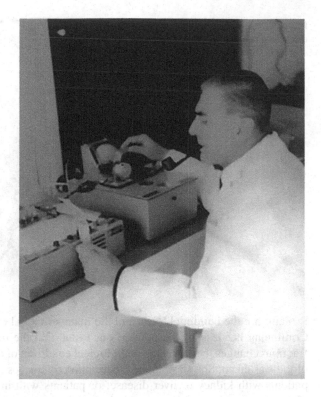

they functioned. After several days of observing how the lab operated, I noticed some small glass slides the doctor was examining with care. I asked Olga what they were. She quite happily sat down at the other microscope, and, like the good teacher she was, she began to explain what she saw to me. The slides were smeared with blood. She showed me the various types of blood cells that circulated in human blood—white and red blood cells and cellular parts, called platelets. With kindness and patience she focused my attention on blood smears from patients, whose cells, particularly their red blood cells, were hosts to foreign bodies. "These blood cells have been infected by malaria parasites," she pointed out to me. After this amazing experience, I spent many days studying glass slides with blood smears (Photo 2.2). To further familiarize myself with these blood smears, I was allowed to borrow a Hematology Atlas from the laboratory's small library. This was great fun and the experience opened new horizons for me and lifted my spirits.

After my introduction to blood smears, my instructor Olga felt it was time to show me a recently developed laboratory technique: the electrophoresis unit. The apparatus had just been brought there by Dr. Achilleas Maroufof, after a short training period in France. "With this device," she told me, "under the influence of its electric field, the proteins contained in blood, depending on their electric charge, move about individually and are separated into five or six major fractions." With those simple words, she explained to me an important area of laboratory and clinical medicine.

Photo 2.2 Author at the
microscope studying blood
smears

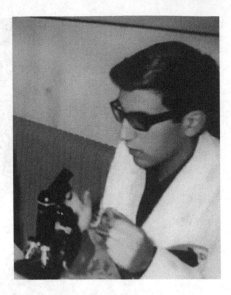

Proteins are the building blocks and the main structural components of our bodies. Continuing her lesson, she pointed out to me that the morphology of the protein fractions changes, based on the pathological condition of the person from whom the blood was taken. She showed me electrophoretic images of the blood samples from patients with kidney or liver disease, or patients with infections. It was fantastic. Those pictures ignited the imagination of this unschooled novice. "With chronic pathological conditions," she emphasized to me, "the γ-globin fractions increase tremendously." Many years later, I realized that this is where the main defensive proteins of an organism, the antibodies, are located. Without knowing it, I had just had my first lesson in immunology.

The laboratory director discreetly kept an eye on my activities. He heard my questions and listened to the answers of the lab assistants. When he didn't agree with the answers or explanations they gave me, he interrupted the conversation and generously gave his own expert opinion. After some time had passed, I don't remember how much, he called me to his office. It was clear that I had earned his trust. He wanted to share his love of research with me.

With a few clear and forthright remarks, he described to me the biggest public health problem in our region. It was brucellosis, that is, a sickness that is transmitted from goats and sheep to people through their unpasteurized milk or through contact with a person with infected animals. His greatest wish, his most passionate scientific pursuit, I would say, was to be able to create a vaccine that would prevent the transmission of this sickness from animal to man. The vaccine would protect the stockbreeders from the infection. But the Brucella bacterium is very crafty. It enters and hides inside the cells of the immune system of humans. Thus, our bodies' defense mechanisms cannot neutralize it. The doctor wanted, with a vaccine, to deter access of that microorganism to its hiding place. Toward this end, he cultivated bacteria.

They would multiply in the culture medium and, in this way, he had at his disposal large quantities of bacteria. Next, he would kill the bacteria by boiling them, and finally he would separate the extracts of the boiled bacteria, through a centrifuge, into fractions. He would take those fractions and administer them to guinea pigs, and he would examine their blood to see if they had developed antibodies against the bacterium. Next, he would test whether the guinea pigs that had developed anti-bodies against the Brucella bacteria were resistant to particular bacteria, which he administered to them in different quantities. This was steady, persistent, meticulous work lasting many years. I remember the notebooks with the experiments. They were well written, detailed, and had pictures, figures, and charts. Unfortunately, I didn't keep any of these experiment notebooks. It was my first indirect training in keeping a scrupulous researcher's diary about the methods used and the results obtained. But alas, all the doctor's efforts were unsuccessful. In spite of the failures, however, I never saw the researcher in him disappointed, tired, or stressed. He did research for his own pleasure; he never felt anxiety about being published, and he never worried about being successful in competitions for funding his research. The penurious public till supported his passion for research. He was like an artist who enjoys his creations and is not interested in earning money. Achilleas Maroufof's attitude toward life taught me which qualities a researcher should have. From the summer of 1963 until his death, many years after I returned from America, our relationship continued without interruption, with enthusiasm and pleasure.

My daily activities at the hospital were just one side of my summer in Ioannina. Short excursions to the island in the lake—back then they seemed like excursions—or to the hill of Ioannina, with boys and girls my age, were a frequent pursuit. Falling in love was one of the most pleasurable experiences of the summer vacation.

The summer went by quickly, with a wealth of experience in all aspects of life. I returned to Athens to register for the second year of medical school. We quickly began classes and laboratories. The quality was uneven. From complete German-style austerity in the anatomy laboratory, to laxness, but with a very good educational program, in the physiology laboratory.

I quickly organized myself in order to acquire as much knowledge as I could, reading two hours a day, not only the books recommended by the professors, but also classical works, such as Sobotta's book on anatomy, Wagner's on histology, and Houssay's on physiology. My reading was always accompanied by low-playing music. I didn't care what kind of music it was; I liked everything from classical music to Greek folk music.

My comrade-in-arms in these studies and my close friend throughout my life was Panayotis Mavraganis, the child of a middle-class family from Mytilini. His father, Spyros, was a pharmacist, and his mother came from a wealthy family. Panayotis, the last-born of three boys, had taken on, from his student years, the role of head-of-the-household. He kept track of the pharmacy's activities, ordered medications, and tried to get the best price for them. The family kept a close watch on Mr. Spyros, who was kind-hearted, polite, and outgoing. Everyone believed that the income from the pharmacy was being siphoned off by the family of Mr. Spyros assistant. Panayotis family obligations made him behave very maturely for his age. He was very frugal and only very occasionally came with us on our evenings out.

During our exams in June, Panayotis and I reviewed the subject matter together. The material was already familiar to us from studying and homework. We kept company with two very pretty girls, who were in their last year of high school. But their parents did not approve of their flirting and sneaking about. One day the door of our apartment almost broke open. It was the angry mother of one of our two friends. Without losing a minute, we found a hiding place. It was a walnut-wood armoire, a family heirloom belonging to the family of Panayotis mother, Mrs. Kleio. Both girls hid inside it. We opened the door and were faced with the angry mother. "Where is Myrto?", she asked us. We invited her into the apartment. Politely, kindly and respectfully, like gentlemen, we allowed her to look around the apartment. She didn't find the girls, and she left feeling satisfied.

In what I considered to be the most important subjects—physiology and anatomy—my grades were excellent and I had the highest grades of all the students. The oral exams in histology-embryology gave us some good laughs. The story was repeated by students for many years. The professor of that Chair, the son of a well-known professor of anatomy, did not have his father's good reputation and had, moreover, various idiosyncrasies. During examinations he would soak his feet in cold water, while he demanded that his students come dressed in suits in the middle of summer. I wore my father's winter suit. It didn't fit me very well. I almost got a heat stroke. Soon the turn came for our group of five students. Vasilis Mantouvalos was first, and I was last. The professor asked us to examine some histologic preparations under the microscope. The heat, my agitation, and my fear kept me from seeing what kind of tissue was displayed on the glass slide. He allowed us five minutes to study the glass slides, and when the time was up, he asked Vasilis first what he saw. Vasilis responded spontaneously, ignoring the advice we had been given by older students. He answered that the tissues were "swiped from a liver." The professor exploded. "Why, you communist," he said, "What kind of language is that?" Poor Vasilis tried to explain to him that he wasn't a communist. After many attempts he managed to whisper: "I'm the son of the chief of the city police." The professor's reaction was to immediately say "I will report you to the chief for changing sides." That ridiculous scene caused me to relax. I looked again under the microscope and I saw that the glass slide had on it a section of the gall bladder. When my turn came, I answered him the way he wanted me to. My reward followed. I received the highest grade he gave to students, that is eight out of ten. My reward for this distinction was a scholarship from the State Scholarship Foundation and an invitation from the professor holding the Chair of anatomy to serve as his assistant. The difficulties were about to begin.

The summer of 1964 was a repetition of the previous one: working at the Hatzicostas Hospital and partying with friends in the evenings and on the weekends.

Upon my return to university in the fall, the third-year courses were absorbingly interesting since they dealt with pathological human conditions. General anatomical pathology: the key to understanding organ injury in the body due to pathological conditions. Pathophysiology: the course that gives medical students an understanding of the mechanisms that cause disease. Microbiology: the study of microorganisms that could potentially invade the human body and cause infections. Pharmacology: the science that analyzes pharmaceutical substances, their effects, and their side effects on the human body. Some of the instructors had a great talent for passing on knowledge, while others were terribly tiring and boring. I was not a student who particularly enjoyed taking theoretical courses. It was my opinion that classes in large auditoriums were a waste of time. But I actively participated in the laboratory exercises and in the patients' care on the hospital wards and in the outpatient clinics. I used the same methods myself as a teacher of medicine with my own students. I taught and still teach based on examples of actual patients.

That year, I had the honorary position of an unpaid sub-assistant for the Chair of anatomy. But the atmosphere there was not compatible with my personality and character. It was strict, for no particular reason, and there were no scientific discussions, or involvement in research projects. I simply could not understand why that professor would hire honor students as sub-assistants. The job he gave us was that of a guard at student laboratories, or worse. When I think back on all this, I still get upset. Instead of the professor readying a new generation of scientists, the climate in his laboratories was to create puppets, capable only of serving the needs of those in power. But fortunately for me, I was soon delivered from this unpleasant situation.

Often it was pure luck, if not coincidence, that saved me. We had training sessions at the microbiology lab. The experiments they showed us, and which we then had to carry out were all familiar to me, because of my experience at the Hatzicostas Hospital. I paid attention, but my mind and my soul were not in it. I had chosen to sit next to a pretty female classmate. Instead of concentrating on the classwork, I would try to impress her. The young teacher in charge of this class had just returned from Germany, after studies lasting many years. It seems the attention I was lavishing on my classmate was so noisy that the instructor took notice. He reprimanded me and moved me to a front-row seat. The punishment wounded my ego and made me ashamed. After a short period of feigned attention to the instructor, I raised my hand to ask a question. I asked him to explain to us why, concerning the Gram staining he was telling us about, certain microbes were colored blue, the so-called Gram-positive, while others, Gram-negative, were red. Instead of answering, he asked me in return if I knew why. With the pompous air of an expert, I gave him the explanation: "Gram-positive microbes have magnesium ions in their outer membranes, which retain blue coloring, while Gram-negative microbes lack these ions."

From my answer he understood that this was not just an innocent question. He called me an impertinent troublemaker and announced to me that after the lab class, I would have to present myself to the chairman of the department to be punished. Mentally falling apart, I waited for the lab class to finish. I felt like a convict being sent before an execution squad. The dreaded moment arrived. I followed him to the chairman's office. The chairman arrived first, and after that I was called in to his office to apologize and be punished.

Professor Ioannis T. Papavassileiou, the chairman of the Department of Microbiology, ensconced in his deep armchair (Photo 2.3) and appearing quite strict, asked me what offense I had committed. I described the entire incident to him. After my account, he asked me how I was doing with my studies and if there were any courses I

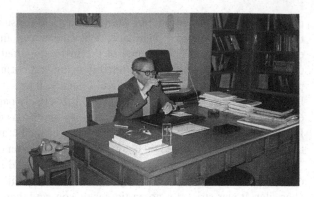

still owed work for from previous years. Cringing, I told him that I had no incompletes in previous courses and that I had a state scholarship. The scene changed completely. He asked me where I had learned so much about microbiology. I described my experience at the Hatzicostas Hospital in Ioannina to him. And instead of exemplary punishment, he offered me the position of unpaid sub-assistant in his laboratory. I accepted it eagerly. That invitation freed me from the oppressive atmosphere of the anatomy laboratory, and microbiology was, for me, a most pleasant scientific pursuit.

That meeting with Professor Papavassileiou was the single most influential event in my academic career. I am grateful to the lecturer who introduced me to the professor, who became my mentor. And from that teacher, after Dr. Achilleas Maroufof, I came to understand the necessity for the experiment. I developed deep-seated respect for the meticulous programming of experiments, their uncompromising repetition, and the most thorough analysis possible of the results, which leads to an understanding of the physiology and the pathology of any living organism. That mild-mannered academician and teacher had a generosity of spirit, a deep knowledge of the science of his subject, a sweeping education, an excellent command of foreign languages, and empathy for the young on their path to maturity and accomplishment.

The microbiology lab was a place of true democracy. The atmosphere at the laboratory was permissive and encouraging to anyone who wanted to get ahead. We had complete freedom. We had ample opportunities for initiatives to do whatever experiments we wanted. It was at that laboratory I decided once and for all that immunology was the field I wanted to pursue. That is where the idea that I might become a university professor was born and developed. It was there that I acquired the confidence that I was capable of setting up an experiment, carrying it out and writing a paper by myself. I was proud because in my final versions the professor made very few corrections. I am sure that he too was proud of me. Until his death the professor and I remained like father and son. In the last years of his life, when his illness rendered him unable to express himself, he tried through gestures and facial expressions, and half-uttered words to explain to the ladies taking care of him that I was his best student. He reacted with childish delight whenever I announced some new scientific paper of mine or took him a book of mine to read. After many years of suffering and loneliness—he had been forgotten by all those he had helped—his life ended. I had the sad privilege of delivering the eulogy at his funeral.

The third year went by nicely. I passed my exams in June. And I went back to Ioannina again in the summer. The Hatzicostas Hospital was there waiting. But my time for scientific pursuits that summer of 1965, the time I devoted to my medical education, was divided between the internal medicine wards and the clinical pathology lab.

I worked alongside a talented clinician, Dr. Lazaros Pouloyiannis. From him, I learned the main nosological entities of medicine: cardiac and respiratory failure, causes of upper and lower gastrointestinal bleeding, pneumonia, meningitis, acute cardiac arrest, snakebites, and finally, in the specially arranged darkened room, I came up against the frightening picture of patients suffering from tetanus. My great desire to become a physician has kept all these experiences intact in my mind. Whenever I encountered something new, I consulted the *Merck Manual for Diagnosis and Therapy* and read up on it. The frightful picture of tetanus sufferers has stayed with me.

That summer, when I was first exposed to the mysteries of disease, I had substantial help from the nurses. They were all notable for their desire to serve their patients and for their kind-heartedness, and they were always ready to teach others whatever they knew, whether theoretical or practical. It was there that I learned to administer all kinds of injections, and there, with their help, that I first inserted nasogastric and urinary catheters, and there that I first took a bone marrow sample. I worked again with most of those nurses when I returned to Ioannina as a professor of internal medicine. They forgot that they had been my teachers. With great enthusiasm and exemplary respect, they worked with me to turn the internal medicine department of the Hatzicostas State Hospital into a university department.

In Dr. Achilleas Maroufof's laboratory, he and I tried to develop a method to study tetanus antibodies in the blood serum of individuals from Epirus. I wanted to see what proportion of the Epirote population was unprotected against tetanus. Our findings would be guidelines for public health services to vaccinate the unprotected. In my efforts to develop this method, I ran into many problems. Only many years later, after I returned from my postgraduate studies in America, did I manage to perfect this method.

During that same summer vacation, I had the good fortune to work with two very interesting volunteers: a German medical student named Ulrich Loss (Photo 2.4), and a young physician serving his obligatory time in the army, Costas Vradelis. Our collaboration was very fruitful, and the advancement of our progress in learning even more so, because we complemented and inspired each other toward the mastery of knowledge. I met both of them again many years later. Ulrich was a well-known professor and researcher in the immunology of the thyroid gland, in Ulm, Germany; and Costas was the director of the Department of Orthopedics in the hospital of the city of Drama, in Macedonia.

My fourth year of studies in medical school was easy and pleasant. All the courses were in clinical medicine, so I had a lot of free time for research in the

Photo 2.4 Author with
Urlich Loss and nurses at the
main entrance of
Hadzicostas Hospital

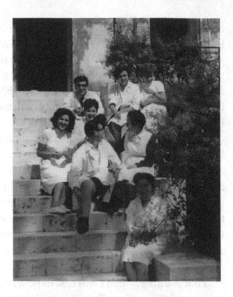

university microbiology lab. That year, I compared different methods for diagnosing pregnancies.

In addition to the classwork, the studying, and the research, a necessary part of our life was also to have fun. My comrades on nocturnal forays were my cousins Giorgos Moutsopoulos and Costas Farmakis. Giorgos, an economist and a high-level manager at the Public Telephone Company, was passionately and devotedly involved in the Movement for Change, promulgated by Andreas Papandreou. He held important positions in government, such as secretary general in different districts of Greece and also in a number of ministries, and as the chief administrator of various organizations. After the government changed, he was obliged to leave these offices, and he did so modestly and without a single illegal drachma in his pocket. Costas works as a lawyer, with a strong sense of ethics and responsibility.

Also inseparable members of our group were: Yiannis Tentes, who served as attorney general for the Supreme Court, highly respected by his colleagues for his knowledge, his ethics, and his contribution to the Greek justice system; Suhel Abu-Gazale, a Palestinian, first-rate medical student, who is a professor of emergency medicine in the U.S. state of Alabama; and the artist Giorgos Papanikolaou, who is no longer with us, the victim of the high speeds he loved. The group was graced by the presence of lovely-looking women. We had discovered a small nightclub in Plaka. The woman who sang there, Yiota Yianna, had a fantastic voice. We went there often. We enjoyed Greek folk music and when we were feeling in particularly high spirits, we would get up and dance. Entertainment, however, was never at the expense of my medical studies. We did it in our spare time.

That year, with a large one-time payment he received when he retired, my father bought a spacious apartment in the neighborhood of Ambelokipoi in Athens. Male and female students from Ioannina used to meet there. On occasional evenings, the student gamblers would gather there, led by my brother, and play cards for hours. I never joined them. I was not excited by the idea of sitting for hours in a chair. Today I use this apartment as my medical office.

In June of my fourth year of medical school, I got a failing grade in my exams for the first and last time. Some of the chaired professors engaged in the unethical practice, with the help of their publishers, of keeping a list of the students who bought the textbooks they had authored. One such person was the professor of radiology. In reaction to this practice, which went against my beliefs, I performed the following experiment: I didn't buy my professor's textbook but instead bought an English text-book on radiology. I used that book to study for my exams. The professor examined us in person. The students were called to be examined ten at a time. My turn came. From what I can remember I was fifth or sixth in line. The exams were monitored by the docent (a position more or less equivalent to that of assistant professor) of that Chair. He served as an usher of sorts. From the questions the professor had asked the students, it became clear that the proper procedures for determining grades had not been followed. The questions to some students were standard, for others they were different, and for still others, those condemned to fail, they were impossible. I was one of the "condemned," seeing as my name was not on the list sent to the professor by his publisher. He asked me if I knew the cause of sarcoidosis. I answered him with certainty that it was a disease of unknown causes. And that, moreover, is still true today, sixty years later. He answered that this is not what he said during class. "I know that," I told him, and continued: "You said that sarcoidosis is due to the toxin of Koch's bacillus." I had the gall to further tell him that his opinion was wrong, and I went on: "If what you said were true, then patients with sarcoidosis should be positive when given a Mantoux skin test, but they are all negative." He lost his temper and ordered the docent to throw me out. For the first time in my student years, I got a grade of zero. I took his exams again in September and was well prepared, but as soon as my turn came, without examining me, he sent me out of his office with a grade of three and told me disdainfully that I would never pass his exams. But in the December exams, which were written exams graded by a committee, the digit 1 was added before the 0, and I got the highest grade, that is, ten. And so my self-esteem was restored and, most importantly, I kept my scholarship from the State Scholarship Foundation. Many years later, the son of that radiology professor happened to be a student of mine. He was a withdrawn young man, well dressed, very serious for his age, an introvert, and a loner. I tried, as best as I could, to help him advance his medical knowledge. I don't know what became of him in life, nor did I ever find out if his father realized that his son's professor at the Medical School of Ioannina was the same young student whose life he had once made so difficult.

That summer, when the fourth year had finished, I stayed in Athens for two reasons: the first was that I fell madly and deeply in love, and the second was the experiments at the microbiology laboratory at Athens University. But I missed having contact with patients. I needed to find a private hospital to work in. Practically next door to my apartment, in Ambelokipoi, was the Asklipeio Hospital of Athens, a good-sized private hospital in those days. I found out that they were hiring medical school students. I decided to meet with the director of the hospital, Dr. Prouskas. I asked for an appointment for an interview, and they gave me one immediately. He was a rather stout, middle-aged gentleman whose dress and pronunciation resembled that of emigrants repatriated from America. I described my experience at the Hatzicostas Hospital, in Ioannina, and told him I was looking for work. His face lit up with a broad smile. "We're from the same place," he told me, most pleased. He hired me as an afternoon doctor without a degree, in the position of a male nurse.

I worked afternoon and evening shifts, every other day. I was paid 3,000 drachmas a month for this work. Quite a good income for those days. I was the most prosperous of all my fellow students. With this income from my work and my scholarship, I furnished our student apartment, was able to purchase foreign medical textbooks, and relieved my family of the financial burden of my living expenses.

The medical and social experiences in that hospital were unforgettable. I came into contact with excellent teachers. I will mention two of them here: Professor Giorgos Merikas and Dr. Nikos Salesiotis. The latter taught me about electrolyte regulation and acid–base balance. He was an excellent general surgeon and a sharp-minded diagnostician. I dealt with cases covering the entire gamut of medicine. I also had the opportunity to handle cases of chronic kidney disease, because the hospital bought a dialysis machine. We operated it with a German doctor, who came to train us. I continued to work in that hospital for the remainder of my student years, as well as during the time I was in military service. This was another important part of my "extracurricular" medical education.

During my last two years of medical school, I became interested in two other medical specialties. It was difficult to decide if I should switch to one of these two fields and abandon my first love, that is immunology. One of my fellow students, Mihalis Manolas, who was quite a bit older than me, worked to make ends meet as a first aid male nurse at the Greek Red Cross, on 3rd September Street. I worked with him many evenings there as a volunteer. Together we treated wounds, inserted catheters, and took care of patients with serious medical problems. I was very interested in surgery. I mulled over the prospect of becoming a surgeon. The results of this specialty are very impressive. The patient arrives in bad health and the surgery returns him to society whole and hearty. Surgeons do not have to deal with the misery of chronic illness. They generally see smiles and expressions of gratitude on the faces of the patients whose problems they have solved. On the other hand, surgeons do not share the other joys of medicine: treating the patient as a whole person—psyche, studying the system affected, and the effects of the illness on the other organs of the body. They miss out on the joy of solving difficult diagnostic puzzles, and they don't have much time for research. So they miss the satisfaction one gets from an experiment and the production of new knowledge. After quite a bit of thinking, I rejected the idea of becoming a surgeon.

The other specialty I fell in love with was psychiatry. I was quite taken by Freud's books. It was gratifying for me, when I had the chance, to try and delve into the hearts and souls of my patients. I realized from a young age that many organic problems people had, were caused by disturbances in their psyche. I was intimidated, however, by a serious lack in my education. I believed that, in order to become a good psychiatrist, you had to have a wide knowledge of sociology, folklore, and philosophy. I had no background in these subjects. I could not foresee then that psychiatry would evolve into biological science. So, with a heavy heart, I renounced that passing infatuation and returned to the folds of immunology.

My final clinical education was in pediatrics, in an up-to-date, well-organized department with all pediatric medicine sections, such as infectious diseases, hematology, gastroenterology, and oncology. This was all due to the administrative talent of the professor and chairman. He was young, eager to work, and exacting, with an excellent education in America. His name was Nikos Matsaniotis. The supervision of the students by the attending physicians was also excellent. My sound background in medicine ushered me easily into the channels of this closely related field. I became good friends with Yiannis Karpouzas, the attending physician of our team, an impassioned lover of medical education, and of the other sex. Or so he liked to boast. I persuaded him to work with me on a study of the epidemiology of toxoplasmosis in children, by studying their reaction to skin tests. That study supplemented the information I had collected from my studies of adults of all ages from different regions of the country. We published the study together.

Just when things were going well, I suddenly began to feel extremely weak. My urine became darker, my temperature went up, and I had no appetite. The diagnosis: hepatitis contracted from blood serum, that is, hepatitis B. I was paying the price for my research. It seems that one of the blood sera I examined at the university microbiology lab was infected. My ailment confined me to bed. The days passed; my skin and my eyes became more and more yellow. The bilirubin in my blood rose to very high levels. My physician, Iraklis Filis, did his best. He gave me corticosteroids and in a few days it all cleared up. Nowadays, this therapy is not recommended and is rather harmful in the case of acute hepatitis B. But two things were worrying me: first, whether my absence from my education at the Department of Pediatrics would be excused, and what punishment I would receive from Professor Papavassileiou. My mind still retained his stringent orders: "If someone gets an infection at the laboratory," he would say, "he should not be allowed back in." Fortunately, however, neither of my two fears came to pass. The Department of Pediatrics did not count my absences and my professor, rather than punish me, stood by me during this trying time.

When I had recovered from hepatitis, I had to help my close friend Panayotis Mavraganis make a desperate wish come true. He was madly in love with Mina Chronaiou, an exceptional student and a serious, modest, and beautiful woman. She was not one to fool around with fellow students. She had been taught at home that to go out with a man meant that she would be devoted to him for life. After some hard thinking, I found a solution: "We'll pay her a visit at home," I told him. "You'll find a way to tell her your feelings there and you'll ask her out." The plan was put into action. I kept Mina's mother, Mrs. Katerina, busy, and the coast was clear for Panayotis to stammer out his passion to the daughter. Everything happened very quickly. In a short time, they were married. It has been over fifty years now. Panayotis, a radiologist, and Mina, a clinical pathologist, enjoy a highly respectable social standing and a substantially successful family: both of their children are physicians. Their daughter Clio devotedly followed everything I taught her and is now a professor of rheumatology at the Athens University Medical School. Their son Dimitris, who is also my godchild, did not succumb to academic pressure. He specialized in radiology. He succeeded Panayotis at their diagnostic laboratory. Panayotis is now a grandfather, crazy about his granddaughter Mina and grandson Kyriakos, Clio's children, and also about Dimitris children, his grandson Panayotis the Second and his granddaughter Melina.

That June, I passed all the required exams and earned my diploma in medicine cum laude. At long last I held a degree in medicine all my own. I still remember my father's telegram:

May God grant you health, strength and the patience to minister to human suffering. May you never neglect to examine your patients from head to toe, regardless of their position, their financial situation or educational level.

Your father Michalis.

Chapter 3
Young Physician

3.1 In the Army

After graduating from medical school, young, male physicians had two obligations: to serve in the army for two or two and a half years, and then to serve in the public health system, by working as a physician in a rural district.

I enlisted in the Air Force in July 1968 to complete my military service. I had no time to waste. I wanted to be finished as soon as possible with my obligations to my country and go abroad to begin my specialization in internal medicine.

At that time, Greece was ruled by a military junta. My first few months in the military training camp were difficult. Every afternoon they called me over the loud-speaker and told me to present myself to the security office of the military camp. The officer in charge, a lieutenant, would give me a good talking to. They wanted to be sure I was not an "enemy of the state," and that I was not an envoy of the "evil powers of the enemies of our country from the north," that is, the communist countries.

There were two things that were not in my favor: my father's record, which was on file in the National Security Office. He was accused of being a communist sympathizer. The man they described was someone other than my father. My father was a democrat, an exemplary and conscientious public servant, a man with the highest moral values, a deeply religious Christian, a very well-educated individual, and a worshipper and servant of the earth and its products. But there was one thing that was true: my democratic father did not sign a declaration renouncing his left-wing beliefs. He did not renounce communism.

The second thing, aside from the "original sins" of my father, was my own record. My father's record made mine worse. First, because I was a member of the Democratic Organization of Epirote Students, and second, because I did not cooperate with the Junta. In the fall of 1967, the government of the Junta had decided to create "fake" student organizations. They selected the students with the best records and appointed them presidents of various university schools. This decision affected me too. I was called in for questioning twice, the first time at the Security Police on Alexandra Avenue, in Ambelokipoi, and the second at the headquarters of the notorious Security

© The Author(s), under exclusive license to Springer Nature Switzerland AG 2022
H. M. Moutsopoulos, *Passion for Excellence*, Springer Biographies,
https://doi.org/10.1007/978-3-031-14128-7_3

Police on Bouboulina Street, behind the Polytechnic School. They announced to me that the dean was going to appoint me president of the medical school student body and they informed me that, if I refused, I would be sent to a "lovely place by the sea." I discussed this with my father, as I always did when it was something important. After thinking for a minute or two, he said to me knowingly: "You could use some rest. You've never gone on a vacation. It wouldn't be all that bad if they sent you for a free vacation on an island." The idea of exile on an island was awe-inspiring. Perhaps it brought back my childhood experiences. But I was terrified at the idea of having to interrupt my medical studies. I decided to follow the advice of my mentor, Professor Papavassileiou: "Let them appoint you and then do nothing." A month or two after my appointment, they fired me because I did not carry out their orders, and they did this after frightening me and putting me through considerable mental anguish at Security Police Headquarters on Bouboulina Street. My short-lived acceptance of this appointment, however, tormented me for many years. I blamed myself for not reacting more forcefully, as I had done so many times in my life.

As a new recruit, I was obliged to do my basic training twice before they sent me for military-oriented medical training. During my second stint of basic training, I was demoted to the rank of soldier without degree. My medical degree was not recognized by the Army. I worked in the administrative office, serving coffee. After a personal and determined intervention by my father, who spoke to the head of the Air Force, my troubles were over. They transferred me to the General Air Force Hospital for two months of training. They appointed me to the internal medicine department. The director of the department was the internist-gastroenterologist Haralampos Bysoulis, a good-natured man eager to communicate and teach his younger colleagues.

Those two months passed quickly. My next transfer orders were for Lefkada, as a physician for the Air Force Radar Station. My duty at the military camp was only in the morning. I had a lot of free time. I rented a spacious apartment on the top floor of a private house on a central street, in Lefkada. My landlord, a kindhearted native of Lefkada, had a shop on the ground floor. He did everything he could to make my stay as pleasant as possible. My apartment was soon transformed into a physician's office. I decided to work afternoons as a general practitioner. At first the office was empty. My main occupation was studying and writing up unfinished papers with the results of my experiments, done at the university microbiology laboratory. But a chance occurrence changed everything. I remember, as though it were today, that one afternoon one of my neighbors, who made and sold salami, came upstairs and, very worried, asked me to go with him to a nearby village to see his sister. "Hurry," he said, "I'm going to lose my sister."

I grabbed my doctor's bag and followed him. My doctor's bag, in addition to the necessary medical instruments (stethoscope, reflex hammer, ophthalmoscope), had all the medicines for emergencies. In a few minutes time, we arrived at the village. It was only a few kilometers away from Lefkada. Outside the house the whole village had assembled, men and women with their children, standing there silently and sadly. I went to the room where the sick woman was. I saw a beautiful, young Lefkadian woman curled up on a couch, the muscles in her face contorted in what looked to me like a neurotic episode. After examining her I explained to her that her life was not in danger, I gave her an injection with a tranquilizer, and got ready to leave. Before I left, I asked them: "Why is the whole village assembled here for such a minor problem?" "A strong and hardy young man," they answered, "is dying in the next room. They just brought him here from the Hippokrateio General Hospital in Athens, so that he could die at home."

I asked them what was wrong with him. They answered that the problem was his kidneys. I got their permission to examine him. We went into his room, where a strong smell like that of a rotten apple hit my nose. That's how chronic kidney sufferers smelled. I went up close to him. He had Kussmaul breathing: short, deep breaths followed by respiratory pauses until they began again. His forehead was full of uremic frost: the accumulation of crystallized urea on the skin. His heart, when listened to, had the sound of intense pericardial rubbing. He was barely able to communicate. I noticed, however, that his urine collector bag was full of urine. I asked them how often they changed it and they answered "twice a day," which means that his urine output was more than three liters a day. With complete certainty I informed them that I could take charge of his case, and that he wasn't going to die. I took the relative who had brought me there with me to Lefkada, where we purchased fluids, electrolytes, vein cannulas and needles. I calculated, without the aid of a laboratory, how much water, sugar and electrolytes I should give him through his veins every day. I stressed to them that they had to carefully measure his urine output, and the intravenous fluids and the liquids they were giving him through the mouth, if he was able to drink. In three days Ilias, the well-known, hardworking porter with the refurbished motorbike, was on his feet and feeling better. I immediately sent him to the nearest hospital to begin hemodialysis.

That incident changed the picture at my office. It filled with patients. I saw everything, from really serious medical conditions to people who just came there to meet me. I never asked them for a fee. But everyone left a little something. In the evening, the right-hand drawer of my desk was filled with money.

My stay in Lefkada will remain in my memory as an unforgettable time. Hardly any patients to see in the morning in the camp, but a lot of studying and writing; and in the afternoon until late in the evening, patients visiting my office. And at night, going out and having fun with other rural doctors my age also completing their obligatory year of public health service in nearby villages.

One night, however, an innocent outing almost cost us very dearly. We were in Nydri, at a small nightclub with bouzouki music and good food. After consuming a good amount of liquor, the dancing began, along with the traditional throwing and breaking of plates. The happy atmosphere was unceremoniously interrupted by the local police sergeant. He had been notified that some young people were breaking the laws against indecent behavior by carrying on like "teddy-boys." He collected us all like so many sacks and hauled us to the police station. He placed us under arrest and opened a case file on us and, in spite of our protests, he sent us before the district attorney. But public opinion in Lefkada saved us. The district attorney issued an order of acquittal.

As a young adult, I was often tormented by sexual longings. In spite of these often overwhelming needs, my productivity concerning studying and learning new things continued to increase. I will not attempt to name all the women I became enamored of. But one woman stood out: Lambrini, the beautiful and intelligent, well-educated daughter of a prominent family from Ioannina, who soon became my girlfriend and eventually my wife and the mother of my children. Her visits to Lefkada were few and far between. She needed to find all sorts of excuses to get away from her house. Her strict mother did not allow her to go out without a reason. So, I had a lot of time for my work as a physician: studying, writing scientific articles and—why not?—entertainment.

After six months on duty at the radar station, new transfer orders came for Tatoi, the major Air Force base in Athens. Two Air Force schools were operating there. One was training officers to become either pilots or airplane engineers, and the other was educating non-commissioned officers in different specialties.

My colleagues in the city of Lefkada had arranged for this to happen in order to get me out of their way. They hoped that by doing this, their own doctors' offices would again fill with patients. With my earnings from office visits in Lefkada I bought myself a small Fiat 850. To me it felt like a Porsche.

In Tatoi, I was placed, as an officer, in the medical branch of the school preparing non-commissioned officers. The director of medical services was a physician, Captain John Kostis. I quickly discerned the depth and the breadth of his knowledge in all specialties of internal medicine. But unfortunately, his stay at the medical office was very brief. He asked for a short leave for training in America and never came back. Today he is professor and chairman of the Department of Cardiology at the Rutgers University Medical School, in New Jersey. He was replaced as director by First Lieutenant Giorgos Terzoglou, an affable colleague with little interest in administration and a friendly, low-key personality that belied his military vocation.

Following a written request by my mentor Yiannis Papavassileiou, I was given permission to leave the camp after the morning office visits, to work as a researcher at the university microbiology laboratory, in Athens. I wanted to finish my experiments for my doctoral thesis. I was studying the epidemiology of tularemia in Greece, an infectious disease spread by bacteria to humans after contact with a rabbit. For that purpose, I would first examine the blood samples for the presence of antibodies against the bacteria, and then I would test the delayed hypersensitivity against the tularemia bacteria by doing a skin test on individuals belonging to different age groups and sexes from different regions of Greece.

At the Air Force camp in Tatoi, aside from my medical duties, I also planned and executed a research project. I wanted to determine whether a skin hypersensitivity reaction to penicillin was a more accurate indicator of penicillin allergy than a previous history of allergy to penicillin in an individual. At that time, there was no such thing as an ethics committee. So, the study went forward without informed consent or ethics approval. I took a detailed medical history of each young man for sicknesses and allergies and followed up by having him undergo a skin test. One morning, during the process of skin testing, a young man, almost six feet tall, after the application of an endodermic penicillin injection, in the space of just a few minutes, collapsed onto the ground. I ran over to him immediately. He had turned blue, was covered in sweat, and had a weak pulse and extremely low blood pressure. I inserted a vein cannula as quickly as I could and began to give him large quantities of normal saline solution, and also a large dose of cortisone, and a small dose of adrenaline. It was only a few minutes until he began to recover. His color returned to normal, his pulse grew stronger and his blood pressure began to slowly rise again. I put him in an ambulance and accompanied him to the Air Force General Hospital. Fortunately, the internal medicine department, where I had worked, was on duty. They welcomed us with kindness and after hearing what had happened, they took charge of all further treatment and hospitalization. I was relieved, and with a weight off my shoulders, I returned to the Air Force camp in Tatoi.

At the camp at Tatoi, I was on duty about once a week. One morning, one of the brighter male nurses, a carpenter in civilian life, called me to examine a student from the Air Force School with a problem that had arisen in the pretibial area. There was a red, raised patch of skin that seemed ready to pop when touched. I asked the young man about it, and he told me it was itching badly. Aside from local discomfort, there was no other problem. If I remember correctly, he was from the lowlands of Thessaly, from a swampy region, and he had only just returned from there a few days earlier, after going on leave. I took a photograph of the diseased skin area and decided to open it and see what was inside. Under the skin, in the subcutaneous tissue, I was met with a surprise. I found a diaphanous sac that had water inside and a worm that looked like a piece of white thread. I opened the cyst carefully and removed the worm. It was quite a novel experience. I placed the foreign body in a piece of gauze dabbed with a normal saline solution, and I carefully cleaned the wound. I didn't sew it up. I let it heal by itself. The young man informed me that he felt better already.

Full of enthusiasm, I took my discovery to go and discuss it with a specialist. And where would the most natural place to go be, if not the Air Force General Hospital? I knew that at the university microbiology laboratory there was no parasitologist. "I'll take it to the director of the dermatology outpatient clinic," I thought, "to Dr. Stefanos Papageorgiou." He was a courteous and unusually well-educated dermatologist who had studied in England. And one, two, three, there I was in his office. I described the patient's problem to him, explained what I had done, and showed him my booty. He looked at me skeptically and, asking himself more than me, he said, "Could this be a yarn from the gauze you used to clean his skin?" "No," I said. "It's a worm that was inside a cyst. I'll take it to Nikos Tzamouranis," I told him. "He's the specialist in parasites at the Hellenic Pasteur Institute." "I think you're making the right decision," he told me. A short while later, thanks to my new set of wheels, I was at the Pasteur Institute. That doctor, a highly astute scholar of microbiology, had never acquired a university title, not even that of docent. The faculty members of the Athens Medical School had rejected his thesis, because it was written in Demotic Greek. The doctor took the worm, placed it on a glass slide, and examined it under the microscope. Immediately, he exclaimed: "This is very rare, it's one of the few times I've seen such a parasite in Greece."

After studying the morphological characteristics of the worm, he decided that it was an undeveloped female Dirofilaria Conjunctiva. "What part of the soldier's body did you find it in?", he asked. "In the pretibial area," I told him. "That location is also rare," he said. "It's a human heteroparasite that's transmitted through a flea-bite. Let's describe it." He took a photograph of the parasite and then took more after staining the Dirofilaria. When I read the bibliography carefully, I saw to my satisfaction that the therapy for this parasitic disease is simply the opening and removal of the cyst containing the parasite. I cannot describe the joy and validation I felt. I went back to Professor Papageorgiou with the results. He was full of admiration for these findings. In a very short time, we wrote up the whole case and sent it off for publication, along with the photographs. The answer from the American *Journal of Infectious Diseases* hit us like a ton of bricks: "We do not accept articles from countries that do not have a democratic system of government." How ironic, I thought. The country that helped abolish democracy, by supporting the military Junta in Greece, is now giving us lessons in democracy. We lost no time and submitted our paper to the journal *Archives of the Pasteur Institute.* It was accepted with praise.

One of the occasional services I had to perform during my military service was that of "inspector physician." That is to say, we examined the suitability of the medicines that had been prescribed, and of the tests that were ordered for the illness of an officer, or his family members. A patient's health booklet had to be submitted to the inspector physician within forty-eight hours from the time the doctor's prescriptions were written. One day, the male nurse on duty showed me a health booklet with a prescription that had been ordered fifteen days earlier. In the place where the inspector physician had to sign, they had already stamped it with the department seal and with mine. With a smile, the male nurse informed me that the stamp had been put there by the officer who owned the health booklet, an arrogant young Air Force lieutenant who kept urging him to "tell the doctor to sign it." Not much later a rather short, but self-important, officer appeared in the office in full uniform. He asked to see the inspector. "That's me," I told him. "Sign this and let's be done with it," he told me. Calmly, I informed him that it was not possible to sign prescriptions written fifteen days earlier, because those were the orders specified to me by the Army Medical Department. "I order you to sign," he said to me. "I don't take orders concerning my signature from anyone," I answered. Then he came toward me, ready to attack me. We soon got into a fight. It didn't turn out well for him. I managed to give him a strong punch that knocked him down. He left the office like a general who had just lost a battle. The incident did not end with the fistfight however. He filed a written complaint titled: "Use of force against a high-ranking officer as witnessed by a low-ranking male nurse." The director of our unit, Commander Sotiropoulos, called me to his office. He was a saint of a man, polite and affable, with nothing militaristic in his behavior, and he was quite clearly on my side. Crushed, he informed me that he had to punish me now to avoid something even worse, that is, my being sent before the Air Force Tribunal. He ordered me to stay under house arrest for twenty days, which meant that I was supposed to stay at home after my morning duties. I left the office feeling calm and proud. If I had reported that officer first for his bad behavior, things would have turned out differently. But back then I was not familiar with administrative regulations, and, to be honest, they didn't really interest me.

In addition to serving in the army, I had permission to work in the Athens University Microbiology Laboratory, which I continued to do with success. Then, I received another bit of news. After graduation, young physicians normally had to wait for a long time until their turn came to start their specialization. By exception, however, students graduating from medical school with honors were now eligible to start their specialization immediately as unpaid interns with an afternoon-evening shift. I began my specialization in internal medicine at the Red Cross Hospital. Every afternoon, I paid a careful visit to the patients I was charged with; I wrote down my findings in the patients' medical records, based on the history of the patient I had taken and the clinical examinations I performed, along with the results of the latest tests, and I made notes on my thoughts concerning the diagnosis and treatment of my patients.

But the research bug had gotten into me. At that time, in 1970, there was a large outbreak of cholera in India, Pakistan, and Iran. The Greek Health Service issued an order for the immediate anti-cholera vaccination of all doctors, nursing staff, and paramedics. I wrote a research proposal to study the immune reactions of Greeks after their vaccination. I discussed my proposal with my attending physician Nikos Markakis and convinced him that this was a study worth doing. He agreed with me. Busy as I was, however, with caring for my patients and with my research, I neglected to carry out the wishes and orders of the department's director. That director believed that the main occupation of trainees in the afternoon hours was to copy the medical records in beautifully crafted letters before they were filed away. In other words, he wanted us to be secretaries. One day, I saw in the unpaid specialists' attendance log, conspicuously written in red ink, the following tragi-comical comments: "The director congratulates the unpaid trainees for copying medical histories. Dr. Moutsopoulos has not copied a single patient's record, and if he continues not to do so, he will be expelled from the department." The director's written reproach surprised me, insulted me, and made me indignant. With a red pen, just below the director's comments, I answered him:

"To the director: seeing as my interest in medicine differs substantially from your own preferences, please accept my resignation." My decision caused an uproar in the department. At the behest of the director, I received phone calls from the attending physicians and the director of the hemodialysis unit asking me to please reconsider my decision. But for me the die was now cast. I never set foot in the Red Cross Hospital again, except once, much later, when I went there as a professor at the Athens University Medical School at the request of the doctors in the Department of Internal Medicine to help diagnose a difficult case.

After that experience, I continued my experiments at the Athens University Microbiology Laboratory. I wrote my thesis, which was examined by a committee of professors from the medical school, and I received my doctoral degree cum laude. At the same time, I was studying for the exams of the Educational Commission for Foreign Medical Graduates (ECFMG), which I passed successfully and with a very high grade. I was now more than ready to go abroad.

3.2 Public Health Service

The time had now come to fulfill my next obligation after my graduation from medical school, that is to say, working in a rural district. I chose to serve as a physician in a district of six villages, fifteen minutes away from Ioannina. The main village was called Grammeno. I chose these villages because they were close to the Hatzicostas Hospital. So, I could now comfortably continue my studies on allergies to penicillin. I developed a protocol that required basophils from the blood of a rabbit, penicillin as the allergen, and the serum of the individual to be tested for the presence of IgE antibodies against penicillin. I developed this method by myself. It required many different skills. First, I had to take blood from a rabbit. I did this with a capillary tube inserted into the canthus of the rabbit's eye. That area has many venules. Next, I had to find a way to centrifuge those tiny tubes. I did not have a centrifuge for capillaries. I had to invent something. I put the capillaries in regular tubes. I had dripped wax onto their undersides. So, the capillary tubes, jammed into the wax, stayed in an upright position. After the centrifuge, I took white blood cells. That required an entirely different technique. I had to break the capillary at the exact point that separated white from red blood cells. Next came the incubation of the white cells with the serum of the patient being tested for the penicillin allergy. If the patient's blood serum contained specific IgE antibodies against the allergen, penicillin, then the rabbit's basophils would be degranulated.

I am proud of the photographs I took under the microscope. These photos clearly show the successive phases of degranulation of the rabbit's basophils, when the blood serum of the individual being tested contains IgE antibodies against penicillin.

The calm rhythm of the rural medical center and my research at Hatzicostas Hospital were cut short when I was notified that Lambrini's father, Thucydides Veloyiannis, had been hospitalized for ten days with a high fever at the Blue Cross Hospital, a private hospital on Vasilissis Sofias Avenue, in Athens. It took me quite a few hours in my super, new car to get to Athens. I took a detailed case history, examined him meticulously, looked at the X-rays and the laboratory exams, and decided that in all probability he had a sub-diaphragmatic abscess, above the liver, that is, an accumulation of pus under the diaphragm. In percussion and in auscultation, the right diaphragm was much higher than the left, and the chest X-ray showed a small quantity of air below the diaphragm.

I called in his physician and shared my thoughts with him. I also suggested to him that a good surgeon needed to give an opinion about the patient. I suggested Giorgos Avlamis, one of the best general surgeons in Athens at that time. A consultation was held and a decision was made in a matter of minutes: the abscess had to be opened and drained. I was present at the surgery. Beneath the diaphragm there was a large accumulation of pus. After the surgeon drained it, he examined it to see what the impediment was that had caused this infectious complication. My future father-in-law's gallbladder was full of gallstones. The gallbladder was removed, and afterward it was determined that his bile duct had an ectopic path. With great skill the surgeon performed a reconstruction of the bile duct. The post-operative recovery of the patient was without problems, and his health was soon restored to normal. From that time on, my father-in-law's opinion of me improved. Whenever he had a chance, he would describe my "great medical skills."

My time in the Public Health Service passed quickly. So, in early fall of 1971, I returned to Athens, having fulfilled all my obligations, and I was now fully equipped mentally, spiritually, and scientifically, for my specialization training in the U.S. That's when we made the big decision. After many years of being deeply in love, Lambrini and I were united in the holy bonds of matrimony.

3.3 Trainee in Internal Medicine

In October 1971, I applied for a specialization in America. I submitted all the necessary documents to the program for selecting doctors wanting to specialize in North America. They placed me in Deaconess Hospital, which belonged to the Harvard University educational program for internal medicine specialization. The hospital asked me for three recommendation letters. I suggested three professors. The programs for specialization training in America begin every year on July 1. So, I had seven extra months, before I left, for additional training in internal medicine. I visited the chairman of what was said to be the best-organized university Internal medicine department. I described to him my scientific career up to that point and asked him to hire me as an unpaid trainee-physician before my departure for America. The law that young physicians who graduated cum laude could, by exception, begin specialization immediately was still in effect. He accepted me in his department and placed me under the supervision of an attending physician. That physician was good-natured, quite well read, and entirely devoted to the patients in the hospital.

I began working immediately. I was in charge of a ward with eight patients. My work at that university department was instructive, pleasant, and productive. Another trainee in the same ward was Sophia Drouva, who was also working as a university assistant at the histology-embryology university laboratory. Extremely polite, sensitive, and a classic Greek beauty, she was very serious for her age. She would not let you get away with anything. We became good friends. We met again in San Francisco, me as a resident in internal medicine, specializing in autoimmune rheumatic diseases, and she as a graduate student working toward her Ph.D. in physiology. We had an unforgettable time in San Francisco. Today Sophia is a professor of physiology in Marseille, France. She never came back to Greece. I have not seen her for years. I still miss her.

June was approaching and I hadn't heard a thing from the Deaconess Hospital. I remember that it was the middle of June when I decided to telephone them. They hadn't sent me the necessary papers to get my visa, the DSP-66 certificate. My call was answered by a gentle, female voice in the admissions office. She politely informed me that they had not accepted me into their educational program, because of what the chairman of the Department of Internal Medicine of the hospital where I was working had written. She would not give me any details about the reasons for my rejection. Her answer left me stunned and drained of emotion. It seemed incredible, inconceivable. What followed was anger and unspeakable rage in the face of this betrayal. That same professor, two months earlier, had called me to his office, congratulated me on my scientific progress and offered me the position of a paid resident in internal medicine. I politely reminded him that I had only been in his department for a few months and that I was planning to leave for America, in June. How was it possible that a professor and internationally renowned researcher, a profoundly erudite doctor, with what I believed to be an upstanding character, could do such a thing to a young colleague? I couldn't make sense of it. I never believed that he did it to harm me. In all probability, he forgot to write a recommendation letter and send it.

That afternoon, we had a family conference. My father-in-law, a well-known lawyer, financially independent, extremely clever, with an even-tempered and amiable personality, suggested buying a private hospital. "There's no need for you to struggle," he told me. "We'll buy a hospital and you'll do whatever you like, from research to clinical medicine. You'll be the director." He did not want his only daughter to go abroad. He didn't want her to live far away from them. My father, as always, was the last one to speak. He liked to speak in generalities. He considered the Moutsopoulos men to be a single unit. "We are not cut out to be merchants, dear friend," he said. "Medicine is a profession. Akis," he said, referring to me by my nickname, "must do his specialization training." And turning toward me, he said in a decisive tone of voice: "Take this money for your ticket and another two hundred dollars for expenses until you find work, and leave immediately." He knew only too well what I wanted.

The next morning, without getting permission, I went to the office where the attending physicians were giving their morning reports to the professor and chairman of the department on the patients' conditions. In front of everyone I said to him: "Professor, what you did was neither ethical nor academically acceptable. I'm leaving for America and you can be sure I am going to succeed there." If I remember correctly, he stammered, "And what do you think America is anyway … Athens?".

One of the attending physicians, who was quite fond of me, would remind me, whenever we met on my short return visits from America, about that incident and express his admiration for my courage.

I packed up some clothes, bought myself a ticket, and on June 18, 1972, I was on my way to Washington D.C. on a TWA flight. My decision to go to that particular city was determined by three factors: as someone who came from the provinces, I believed that being in a capital city was the best choice. I also knew that there were numerous medical schools in the area. But the major factor was that Professor Nikos Papadopoulos had arranged for his colleague, Yiannis Kintzios, to pick me up at the airport.

Nikos Papadopoulos was from Epirus. He emigrated at an early age and studied biochemistry in America. He worked in large hospitals in Washington and became a professor of biochemistry at Georgetown University. He had returned to Athens for a short period and was working as the biochemistry director at the National Research Foundation and as a professor at the Athens University Medical School. That is when my mentor, Yiannis Papavassileiou, introduced me to him. Nikos and I had many long scientific discussions. He wanted me to collaborate on his research studies. But my decision had already been made: specialization in America.

It was the first time I traveled by airplane and my first trip abroad, across the Atlantic no less. I was full of enthusiasm to be leaving for specialization in the U.S. Mr. Kintzios was waiting for me at the airport holding a sign with my name written on it. Nikos Papadopoulos had notified him. He was Nikos colleague at Walter Reed Hospital. I felt relieved. He was accompanied by his wife Mary, a gracious lady, who spoke Greek with difficulty and a heavy accent. Instead of taking me to a hotel, they put me up in their house, where a delicious, hearty meal was followed by many hours of sleep. The next morning, I was ready for action.

Chapter 4
Emigrant

4.1 Physician in Training

4.1.1 Washington, D.C.

The next morning, I woke up fresh and raring to go, ready to start searching for a hospital to train at. After a lovely morning with the Kintzioses—they lived in a small apartment in Silver Spring—I asked them to take me, if possible, to a hotel that Professor Papadopoulos had recommended to me. I wanted to gather my thoughts and get moving. My number one priority was to find a job that would give me the opportunity to continue my specialization in internal medicine and take care of my living expenses at the same time. Yiannis Kintzios went to the research institute at Walter Reed Hospital where he worked, and Mary took me to the hotel. It was on Georgia Avenue, near the border between the state of Maryland and Washington D.C. It was a difficult area in which to walk casually in the street or go out at night could be dangerous. The least that could happen to you was losing your wallet. But mine was already almost empty.

At the reception desk of the hotel, a sullen, middle-aged man was seated, busy with his papers. He was dressed like an American, with checkered trousers and a multi-colored shirt. I could tell from his pronunciation that he was Greek-American. I introduced myself and stated the reason for my visit to America. He listened to me half-heartedly. He seemed not to believe what I was telling him. In order to convince him, I opened my doctor's bag—a brown leather bag that was designed and hand-made by my father—and took out my papers. I spread them out on the reception desk. He looked at them carefully. He read them and then the expression on his face changed from indifference to courtesy, and his behavior became almost subservient. He offered to carry my things and led me to my room on the second floor. It was poorly furnished but sparkling and clean. The bedspread was adorned with a tiny hole or two. What could one expect when the room cost only twenty dollars per day?

After the short time it took me to unpack the few clothes I had, I went back down to the reception area. "What can I do for you, doctor?", the receptionist said

H. M. Moutsopoulos, *Passion for Excellence*, Springer Biographies,
https://doi.org/10.1007/978-3-031-14128-7_4

delightedly. "We have to find the telephone numbers of the chairmen of the internal medicine departments at the university hospitals in the area," I told him. He opened the telephone books for Maryland, Virginia, and Washington D.C. and began meticulously looking up the phone numbers. We found about twenty of them. It was time to start making calls. When I first went to America, my spoken English was not very fluent, while I could read and write the language fairly well. I asked him to make the calls himself and speak as though he were me, after having thoroughly briefed him about what he needed to say. He made one call after another. They all gave him the same standard response: "It's too late to hire a physician for specialization, all the positions are taken." But they all suggested that he leave our phone number, in case a position opened up at the last minute.

The first day passed quickly. In the afternoon before he went off duty, Paul Tsakalakis, who was not only the receptionist but also the owner of the hotel, asked me if I had somewhere to go for dinner. I had no other invitation, so I happily accepted his. We drove to his house in his big, long Buick. His house had a very large, well-kept garden, and a huge, four-car garage. As soon as the car came to a stop in the garage, his gracious, well-dressed wife, Maria, appeared. She welcomed us in the manner of an urbane hostess in any provincial city of Greece. Then she led us to the dining room. The table was nicely set and ready with many different dishes and plenty of wine. We sat at the table with their children, Terry and Jimmy. They were about ten years younger than me. They all wanted to know why a doctor from Greece would leave the beautiful climate of Athens and a good social position to come and struggle in America. Was it for the money, perhaps? They could not get it into their heads that a doctor had emigrated to improve himself, to become a better doctor, to increase his knowledge.

The food was delicious. Maria was a classic Greek housewife. Hospitality was in her blood. She had come to America many years before. They had shown her a photograph of Paul, she liked him, so she got on a boat and traveled for fifteen days until she reached America. She raised a terrific family and tried to keep all the Greek ethnic, holiday, and religious traditions. The only thing she changed was her language, but even in English she spoke in another dialect, which can be called "Greek-American" or "Gringlish." She called the refrigerator "friza," the roof of the house "roufi," an automobile "karo," a company "kompania," a contract "kontaki," the hospital "spitali," and so on and so forth. From that day on, Paul and Maria's house became my house too.

Through Maria and Paul, the houses of all their relatives were opened wide to me. Every once in a while, when I had a free Sunday, I enjoyed Greek delicacies in their households. They were all proud of their origins. They urged their children to study hard, while at the same time they worried about how to keep them aware of their Greek-Orthodox heritage. They insisted that they go to Sunday school at the Greek Church every week on 16th Street, in Washington, D.C. What they wanted most was for their children to marry Greeks. Unfortunately, none of them obliged.

A few days later, I received the news I had been so anxiously awaiting. They called me from the office of the chairman of the internal medicine department of Georgetown University Medical Center to tell me that I had an appointment with the chairman on such and such a day at such and such an hour. Unexpectedly, a trainee would not be taking up his position. Thus, there was a vacancy for an intern's position that had to be filled immediately. Paul and I planned how I would get to the hospital in Georgetown. "I'll switch shifts with someone else at work and take you there myself," he told me.

We were right on time for the appointment. The central hospital of the university was located right in Georgetown, the best and most expensive area in Washington D.C. We were soon in the office of the chairman. His waiting room was a large space with secretaries. We told them who I was. Soon afterward, most probably after being notified by his secretaries, the imposing figure of Professor Dudley Jackson, the well-known hematologist and specialist in platelet disorders, greeted me and ushered me into his office. It was the first time I saw a professor not sitting in the armchair behind his desk, but in one of the two chairs that had been placed in front of the desk.

The first question he asked was why I wanted to become an internist. With the little English I knew, I described my experience. I was well prepared. Instead of words, I showed him my medical degree and my doctoral thesis, both the originals and the official translations. I also gave him a packet with thirteen published research papers. I described to him, as best I could, my experience in internal medicine, and I told him with certainty that I wanted to be a clinical immunologist, and in particular a specialist in infections that attack immuno-compromised individuals. I could see conflicting emotions written on his face. It wasn't long before he put them into words. "You look very good on paper, but you don't speak English," he said to me. With confidence, I answered that he could hire me as an unpaid intern, and that all I needed was for him to offer me room and board. "Please give me a chance, try me out," I told him. I think that in spite of my limited English, I made an impression on him. He hired me. He gave me the position of intern in an affiliate of Georgetown University Hospital, the Providence Hospital. Georgetown University Medical School, in order to train medical students and to provide specialization in internal medicine for young physicians, used six hospitals: the Central University Hospital, the Veterans Administration Hospital, Washington General Hospital, Fairfax Hospital, Arlington Hospital, and Providence Hospital.

Fortunately, the hospital provided accommodation to interns and residents, who were in its program for specialization in internal medicine. My roommates were Henry de Silva, from India, and Roberto de Petri, an Argentinian. Henry was a kind-looking figure, somewhat dark-skinned, and rather short. His mobility was seriously impaired due to polio. Roberto was the well-educated, financially comfortable son of a political family from Buenos Aires. He always ate with a knife and fork. For him, meals were a sacred ritual. Henry and I ate standing up, without much fuss. On July 1, we began to work and study toward our specialization. After a short briefing, each of us was placed in a particular section of the Department of Internal Medicine. They gave us the training program for two months and told us emphatically that every evening from six to eight we had special orientation classes about our new duties. In those classes, every section head briefed us on the section's function and our responsibilities. They explained to us how to request tests carried out in a corresponding department, how to write prescriptions, and twice a week we had intensive training in cardiopulmonary resuscitation. Also, twice a week was a class on how to evaluate electrocardiograms, and once a week we had a class on medical ethics and conduct.

The first training position I was assigned to was in the intensive care unit (ICU). When I began work in that unit, I had never seen anything like it. It was like a factory. Machines were everywhere. There were patients lying on cots. Most of them were hooked up to a respirator, and all of them were monitored for their pulse, blood pressure, and electrocardiographic rhythm. We soon heard some bad news. Professor Robert Kelley, the director of the unit, a strict, demanding man of Anglo-Saxon heritage, had an extreme dislike of foreigners. He considered them second-class citizens. A second-year resident was the head of our team, consisting of me and two fourth-year medical students. A stern, upright man of few words, he motioned to indicate that it was time to begin our rounds to see our patients.

We stopped by each patient's bed. Our team leader explained to us the reasons for each patient's admission to the ICU, summarized the clinical and laboratory findings on that particular patient, discussed the progress of the illness, and suggested additional tests or modifications of therapies. At the end of the patient rounds, he urged us to carefully study each patient's record.

When recording the course of an illness in a patient's medical records, we had to strictly follow a certain order: (a) subjective complaints by patients; (b) objective findings from clinical examinations and laboratory results; (c) assessment of the patient's condition based on subjective and objective findings; d) plans and further action. The initials of each stage spelled the word "soap." In other words, using this method on a daily basis, we could get a "clean" view of a patient's condition. I took notes on everything the resident leading the team said. At the end of these initial, instructive medical rounds, I realized that all of my patients were in need of arterial blood gas measurement. This was an entirely new medical procedure for me. I had never had the opportunity to work in an ICU in Greece. There was only one substandard ICU in all of Athens, at the Sotiria Hospital.

I hurried to the hospital library. I opened a book on chest diseases and quickly read the chapter on arterial blood gas. I immediately understood that in order to take blood, I had to puncture an artery. I went back to the ICU and confidently approached a nurse and asked her to show me where I could find the necessary equipment to take arterial blood gas. She quickly opened a disposable plastic case with all the necessary equipment: syringe, needle, and heparin—to prevent blood clotting—as well as gauze pads. Before I attempted to puncture an artery, I asked the nurse: "From which artery do we take blood to be tested?" "The first choice is the radial artery," she said. She cleaned the radial area with antiseptic, prepared the syringe, and gave it to me. I was ready for the procedure. Fortunately, my first attempt was successful. The syringe filled almost completely with blood, which came up with great pressure. "That's enough," she told me. With my mind clouded by the joy of my success, I did not press on the punctured artery as required. Fortunately, the nurse quickly applied pressure there, covering up my mistake.

The work in that unit was demanding, and the hours there were interminable. We were on duty every other day, that is, we would work for thirty-six hours, have a twelve-hour break to rest, and continue working for another thirty-six hours.

Communicating with those patients who were not on respirators was difficult. How could I understand in my overworked state what they were saying? Half of what they said was unintelligible and full of idiomatic expressions. The expectations of our superiors concerning our professional competence and progress were enormous. With the passage of time, I adjusted to the demands of my unit, and my ability to communicate with patients, hospital personnel, and my superiors improved. My relations with Professor Kelley were cool and impersonal. His ability to fill the gaps in our training, add to our knowledge, and stimulate us with the right questions to seek out new things was incomparable.

In addition to the hard work in our unit, the demands of the office of education under the supervision of Professor Harold Weise were rigid and inflexible. Regardless of our workload, we had to take part in all the educational activities of the department. Once a week were grand rounds, that is, departmental clinical pathology discussions of two cases, led by a visiting professor. Also once a week, we had a clinical radiology meeting, where a member of the radiology department, using X-rays, showed us very interesting findings concerning different nosological entities. In that way, our ability to read X-Rays improved rapidly. Once a month was a mortality conference—a discussion of causes of death—which included a rigorous analysis of the causes that led our patients to die, based on post-mortem findings from autopsies. My social interaction with my two roommates was for about one hour every two days. Henry was my English teacher, while Roberto needed psychological support. He couldn't take the pressure. I played the role of his psychologist without a degree. Every time we met, he would tell us that he planned to return to his country. I was in fact a successful psychologist, because not only did he not discontinue his studies to return to his country, but he stayed permanently in America as an internist near Saint George, Maryland. Henry is a professor of hematology at Temple University Medical School, in Philadelphia.

The last day I was on duty at the ICU, Professor Kelley called me in to his office. In a most friendly manner, he congratulated me on my progress and told me that he was impressed by my knowledge and my devotion to my patients. Then came the best part of all. He invited me to his house for dinner. From what I found out later, I was the only foreigner ever to set foot in his house. "I know that you're not on duty," he told me. "I checked the schedule." I was ecstatic and thanked him profusely. "There's only one problem," I told him."I don't have a car." "Don't worry. This afternoon at 5:30 I'll pick you up at the doctors' residence."

The work in the internal medicine team was a piece of cake. With my experience in Greece, I played the role of teacher for my colleagues. Everyone asked for my opinion. In the medical wards, I acquired another skill. I became an invasive internist. My long-buried desire to be a surgeon came to the surface. It was there that I learned how to insert catheters in a subclavian vein, how to take bronchial secretions from patients in a coma by inserting an inter-laryngeal catheter, and how to perform an organ biopsy such as on the liver, the pleura, and the peritoneum.

My English, however, was still a problem. I could barely understand what people said to me when I was on duty. Normally, during those thirty-six-hour shifts, one could find time to relax and even nod off for a bit. But I rarely did this because, for me, my shifts were an occasion to practice my English, especially my listening skills, which were still sadly lacking.

One night the following humorous incident occurred: the nurse on duty called me over to perform what was called "pronounced dead," that is, to sign the death certificate of a patient, who had just died from metastatic cancer. I did not understand this order. I went into the patient's room and, the minute I saw him there dead, I sounded the special emergency alarm known as "code blue," to resuscitate individuals in case of sudden death. The nurse tried in vain to stop me, absorbed in performing the kiss of life and thumping periodically on the dead man's precordium. In a minute, a special team arrived with a trolley containing medicines, electrolyte solutions, needles and syringes, an electrocardiograph, and a defibrillator. But they were unusually indifferent, and instead of taking part in the resuscitation, they were smiling. The team leader pulled me away from my work and, speaking slowly, explained to me that the patient had passed away. In the end, I realized I'd made a blunder.

My difficulties communicating in English were even more apparent during the morning reports. After our shift, at nine in the morning, we had to present a synopsis of the newly admitted patients to the director of education, Professor Harold Weise. Whenever he considered that a case had educational value, he encouraged us to present it in detail. He used the case as an opportunity to teach us about differential diagnosis, how to make a diagnosis, and on what basis to start proper treatment. That physician was profoundly knowledgeable about most nosological entities of all systems and organs of the human body. He was exacting with himself and very demanding of his interns and residents. During the morning reports, he stressed the importance of taking a careful medical history of the patient, and doing a thorough examination of all the patient's organs and systems.

The professor demanded that we examine the eye front to back—and for that purpose I bought a very expensive ophthalmoscope, which cost half of my monthly salary—and also that we perform a complete neurological examination and a manual examination of the rectum and the vagina, in the case of a woman, and that we do this for every patient, regardless of the reasons that brought him or her to the hospital. "By examining many individuals, you will come to know what is normal," he would tell us "and you will understand the pathological when you come across it. Then, when you have formulated your own opinion, you will call the specialist to confirm your findings, and he will suggest specific diagnostic tests and/or therapies. If you don't examine your patients thoroughly, you will never become competent internists, but simply managers of your patients."

When it came to ordering tests, he was quite stingy. He wanted us to justify every test we ordered. He would turn livid whenever we uncritically amassed useless results. He followed the same script for the therapeutic procedures we carried out. Medications were given only when they were strongly indicated. He did not allow us to prescribe any antibiotics that were not on a list of ten he had given us. If we wanted to use a different one, we had to justify our decision. He did have one fault.

He would make fun of the mistakes we made in grammar and pronunciation. I was one of the interns who were particularly targeted by his irony.

I will never forget one of the morning report sessions. I was presenting data on an African-American patient who had a fever and chest pain that interfered with his breathing—we physicians call this pleuritic pain—and during the clinical examination, I had encountered sounds of pericardial rubbing in the pre-cardiac area. The pericardium is the sac that encloses our heart, and the rubbing sound is like that of two pieces of leather rubbing together. With great confidence, in spite of my limited English, I presented my diagnosis, based on the clinical picture, a cardiogram, and a chest X-ray. "Pericarditis, most likely caused by a viral infection," I said. He looked at me ironically and asked, "What is the patient's profession?" "Unemployed," I answered. "What are his eating habits?", he continued. I had no answer to his question. "How much alcohol does he consume every day?" "Five beers," I answered. "Wait, my friend, for the results of the Mantoux skin test for tuberculosis. Then call the thoracic surgeon for a biopsy of the pericardium. Despite the severity of his case, which points to viral-induced pericarditis, I believe he is suffering from tuberculous pericarditis. First, because African-Americans live in unsanitary conditions; second, they are undernourished, and third, your patient is an alcoholic. All those things lead to the weakening of the immune system and the appearance of tuberculosis," he said.

I did all the tests and the professor was right. That taught me a lesson, and I learned that if we want to make a proper diagnosis, we mustn't omit any parameters from our medical thinking. And I learned one more lesson. That professor did not want obedient and subservient co-workers, but mature physicians, who could improve their skills by learning from their mistakes. Once the diagnosis was finalized, he made no comments. But for me, my mistake and the lesson I learned have remained indelibly in my memory.

One morning, several days after I began my training in the internal medicine wards, the secretary of the director of education showed me a glass tube and politely and discreetly asked me if I knew what it was for. Probably because of the bewildered look on my face, she realized that I didn't. She explained to me that we use it on our underarms after bathing. It was a tube of deodorant. It seems that the odor produced from the secretions from my sweat- and sebum-producing glands was creating a problem for my co-workers, and probably for my patients. I was so ashamed I wanted to dig a hole and crawl in. With the little self-esteem still left in me, I thanked her and promised her that I would buy some deodorant and begin using it.

After my two-month stint with the patients in the internal medicine wards, it was my turn to work for a month in the intensive care unit for coronary artery diseases. There, thanks to studying and with the help of the nurses, the chief resident, and the director, I perfected my skills in diagnosing and treating every type of arrhythmia and the complications of heart disease. The head of that unit was Professor Mike Fletcher. He was an internationally recognized expert on cardiac arrhythmias. Painstakingly and patiently, he examined every cardiogram of every patient. With a centimeter ruler, he would measure the electrocardiogram waves and try to teach us which arrhythmia was dangerous and which was not. After the visit, he would meticulously summarize the data from the final minutes of each patient who had died the previous day in our unit. He would check the tapes on the patient's electrocardiographic monitor. He read the notes of the doctors on duty and the nurses about diagnostic and therapeutic procedures performed on the patient. Gently but decisively, he would point out deficiencies in our medical performance and would be delighted like a small child when our actions were flawless.

Training continued. Life went along at the same rhythm: hospital, home, hospital. Too much work and too little food—I couldn't get used to hospital food and when I was home in the evening I didn't feel like cooking—caused me to lose 15 kilos from my already low body weight before I left for America. I had no time to see the families who had befriended me, when I first came to America. If I had managed to visit with them, their delicious home-cooked meals might have added a few kilos to my weight. I wasn't ungrateful, but I greedily spent the limited free time I had to rest and study. Studying was based on whatever incidences of illness I dealt with. My reference book was *Harrison's Principles of Internal Medicine*. It is filled with underlinings in the text and notes in the margins. Six months after the beginning of my specialization, two emotionally charged events occurred. My friend, colleague, and English teacher, Henry, fell seriously ill with a fever and a cough. He was spitting up blood. He was diagnosed with acute pulmonary tuberculosis. Working too hard and eating too little, along with bad quality food, ruined his immune system. He saved as much money as possible, because he sent three quarters of his meager earnings to his family in India. I was very upset, as though a brother had fallen ill. Fortunately, however, his illness responded quickly to the anti-tuberculosis treatment.

The second event in some way balanced out the anxiety I felt during Henry's illness. They called me from Professor Jackson's office and announced that my exile at Providence Hospital was over. They had scheduled me to spend three of the next six months at the Central University Hospital and another three months at the Veterans Administration Hospital. My self-esteem began to grow, based on my skills. This move created two problems that demanded immediate solutions: buying a car and renting an apartment. I went to the bank to take out a loan. I had decided to buy a Toyota Celica. The bank employee explained to me that because of my short stay in America, the bank did not consider me trustworthy. To get a loan, I had to have someone sign as a guarantor.

My friends' credentials did not meet the criteria for the bank. At the hospital where I was working, the director of the training program in obstetrics and gynecology was Dr. Peter Protos. A Greek from Naxos, a specialist in gynecological endocrinology, and an excellent clinician, I thought that he would be the perfect person as a guarantor. I asked Professor Protos' secretary for an appointment concerning a personal matter. In a few hours' time, he called me to his office. I introduced myself to him, and he told me that he had heard about me, adding that he was aware of my good reputation. That calmed me, and easily and without a second thought I said to him: "I want to buy a car, it's an absolute necessity because they have moved me to different hospitals of the medical school. The bank is asking for a guarantor." "Don't worry, we'll get this all worked out by tomorrow," he said. The next day his wife, Efi, brought me a check for the entire amount the car was worth. Very politely and carefully, so as not to make me feel bad, she said: "You can pay us back whenever you're able to."

That car remained my trusted companion during all of my stay in America. Once I had it, I now had to learn the way to the hospitals. After practicing on paper, I took my first exploratory drive, accompanied by Paul Tsakalakis' son, Terry. It wasn't so difficult. At the same time, I started looking for an apartment. After a quick search for safe and affordable neighborhoods within reasonable proximity to both hospitals, I rented an apartment in the Blair Plaza apartment complex, in Silver Spring.

On my first free weekend, I planned a visit to New York to see my cousin Haris Tsoukanelis. We were classmates and friends. We had some crazy times together in Ioannina. When he was still in high school, in the tenth grade, he took some special exams, received a scholarship, and left for America. His purpose was twofold: to fix α congenital ear defect through plastic surgery, and to study. He managed to do both. He became a successful director of a large bank in Manhattan, and with a new earlobe. He gave me precise directions as to which highway to take and where to exit to get into Manhattan. The trip to New York City was a new experience for me. The roads were wide, and the bridges were huge, many of them crossing one over the other. I took it all in with awe and amazement. "Look where I am," I thought to myself, "from my life in poor little Greece to the majesty of America." The weekend in New York was filled with even more excitement: fancy restaurants, Broadway shows, and shopping at department stores I had no idea even existed. With a wealth of new experiences after a fun-filled weekend, I returned to work.

My experiences at the university hospitals in Georgetown were incomparable. I was bombarded with knowledge from distinguished professors. You needed to have antennas to receive all the messages. I remember them all with extreme gratitude. To keep things brief, I will only mention a few: Hyman J. Zimmerman, a liver specialist particularly knowledgeable in all branches of internal medicine; Lilian Reeckan, a diabetes expert, who discovered the C-peptide of insulin; Sol Katz, a well-known pulmonologist and one of the greatest proponents of the study of tuberculosis and sarcoidosis; Proctor Harvey, an eminent cardiologist who invented the well-known Harvey's stethoscope, a triple-headed stethoscope named after him; and Dudley Jackson, who, as I have already mentioned, was a well-known hematology researcher.

The clinical pathology conferences were an absolute feast. Based on the cases we discussed, I gobbled up the analysis of differential diagnosis and documented diagnosis. Those professors had the entire bibliography of medicine in their heads. Another important source of learning was the morning report of the residents to the chairman, or his stand-in. There, along with the presentation of each case, we reviewed all of internal medicine. Those were unforgettable years filled with incomparable experiences.

Those years of training drilled into my head the need for classifying patients' problems, the need for well-documented requests for lab tests, and the need for consideration, based on all the data, of the remaining possible diagnoses. Because of the large number of cases we dealt with, from the most common to the most rare, my medical skills were improving every day.

The frequent repetition of invasive methods honed my skills. During the entire span of our medical training, the words of Professor Zimmerman were always in my mind: "When you make a differential diagnosis, give priority to the more frequent medical problems. The rarer ones are always rare."

I could list many examples, but let me focus on the most characteristic. During one of the morning reports to the chairman, we were all exhausted and pale-faced, after a twenty-four-hour shift with difficult but interesting cases. He fixed his gleaming eyes on us and said: "You're beat. I will summarize the main problems of the patients you admitted to the hospital, and we will determine what further diagnostic and therapeutic intervention is needed for each patient." That rigid, exacting, jittery professor was a person with great compassion and humanity. Quite possibly, the chief resident had given him a report before we did. Addressing the resident in charge of each patient, he asked for details of the clinical and laboratory findings, or the incidents that occurred after the patient was admitted.

He wanted to educate us without tiring us. He also wanted to be sure that the patients would have a first-rate hospital stay, without it being influenced by the strain we were under.

That professor obliged us to develop yet another good medical habit. He insisted that every resident examine the slides with his patient's blood smears, and the urine sediment after it was centrifuged. In this way, instead of learning only theoretically about the morphology of the red and white blood cells and the cylinders in the urine sediment, we would also acquire practical knowledge. By performing a Gram stain on the patients' secretions (sputum, urine), we might recognize the type of microorganism that caused the infection. Based on the identification of the microbe, we could then begin proper treatment.

In the early spring of 1973, Lambrini finally came permanently to America. She had finished law school. She too had come to America in the hope of studying. But there was one problem. She didn't know English. She spoke perfect French, but that was useless in America. The first thing we did was to find a school where she could learn the language. It wasn't long before she began her studies.

The first year of training in internal medicine was coming to an end. The time came for me to sign a contract concerning my second year of specialization in internal medicine. The educational programs at university hospitals keep only three quarters of the interns of the first year to continue to their second year. It is a pyramid-like system, which is to say that if, in the first year of specialization, there are ten physicians in training, in the second year there are seven, the third year five, and so on. So, the renewal of the first-year, specialization contract is not a given. I was among the lucky ones. My contract was renewed for the second year. But this time, it was with one of the central hospitals belonging to the educational system of Georgetown University Medical School. In addition, I was given a very unique opportunity. After a brief discussion, Professor Zimmerman suggested a short-track contract for me, that is, a brief course toward becoming a specialist in internal medicine. My professors felt that my education in internal medicine in Greece was satisfactory. So instead of three years of internal medicine training to acquire the title of specialist, they would allow me to train for two years, at an enhanced pace. This meant that during my second year as a resident, I would work for eight months in the internal medicine wards, two months in the ICU, one month in the coronary artery disease unit, and one month in the emergency room. I was not allowed time to choose work in other subspecialty sections of internal medicine. In those other sections, the workload and the physical exhaustion were much less. I accepted the proposal most happily. I wanted to start my training in clinical immunology as soon as possible. I wanted to have a chance to work in a research laboratory.

At the beginning of the second year of my specialization in internal medicine, I took the Federal Licensing Examination (FLEX) in order to acquire a license to practice medicine. The exams were long, but not difficult. After taking them, I became a regular physician, able to practice internal medicine and surgery, that is, a general practitioner, with a license to practice medicine in all the states in the country except California, with the same status as colleagues who had graduated from medical school in America. My passion for research flared that year. I had by now broken the language barrier. My medical skills were now accepted and recognized by my colleagues and my professors. So, with the relaxed mindset that comes from success, I was now ready to focus my energy on acquiring new knowledge.

In our department wards, we treated many patients with diabetic ketoacidosis— diabetic individuals whose blood sugar was not well-regulated. In these individuals, their tissue, instead of consuming the correct fuel, that is, sugar, produces energy by burning up fat. This results in their blood sugar level remaining high and prevents potassium, an essential electrolyte, from getting into the cells, where it is necessary for normal cell function, and the pH of the blood turns from neutral to acidic. A tried and tested therapeutic approach for those patients was to administer liquids, electrolytes, mainly potassium, and intravenous insulin, until the metabolic imbalance was corrected. To achieve a better therapeutic result, we administered the insulin intravenously rather than subcutaneously, as is normally done with diabetics. After treating many such cases, an idea came to me. Why not administer the insulin intramuscularly rather than intravenously? I discussed my idea with Professor Reeckan. She found it very interesting. Despite my heavy workload, I wrote up a protocol in a matter of days. We would alternately administer intravenous and intramuscular insulin to patients with diabetic ketoacidosis. This comparative therapeutic approach was moving quickly ahead and nearing completion. Unfortunately, however, there were others who had come up with the same idea before we did. While we were enjoying collecting the results of our project, the other researchers beat us to it. One day I saw their results published in *The Lancet*. Their results were in complete accordance with ours. Intramuscular administration of insulin is more efficient and has fewer side effects than intravenous administration. In spite of our obvious disappointment at our failure to publish our results, that study was, for me, a very useful lesson in clinical research.

Midway through my training, I received the most important gift of all. My daughter Niki-Maria was born, on the feast day of the Virgin Mary, November 21, 1973—a beautiful, dark, thick-haired baby doll.

Niki-Maria did two years of nursery school and two years of primary school in America. She also took Greek lessons at the Saint Constantinos School, run by the Greek Orthodox Church on 16th Street, where Lambrini was teaching Greek. Niki-Maria was a hard-working, excellent student. When she returned to Greece,

Photo 4.1 Daughter Niki
with husband Manuel and
children Ares and Daphne

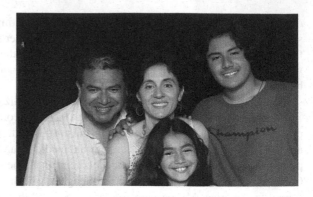

she kept up her English, which she spoke like a native, learned flawless French, while her Greek was the same as that of children her age born in Greece. She passed her exams for university admittance in the school of her choice, for dentistry. When she finished her university studies in Greece, she went back to America, where she was accepted as a research fellow in the immunology laboratory at the National Institute of Dental Research. That was where she wanted to work. At the same time, shortly after she started working there, she began her specialization in periodontics and research toward a Ph.D. I was there in person on the day when she defended her thesis. I was very proud of her. She presented complicated experiments, displayed extensive knowledge of basic science, and answered the examiners' questions quickly and precisely. What else could a father who had devoted his life to understanding human illness wish for? It was the most satisfying moment of my life. Today, she is a renowned immunologist, head of oral mucosal immunology at the National Institute of Dental Research. Aside from her scientific accomplishments, she is married to Emmanuel Osorio, a studious immunology researcher, and they have two, smart, good-looking, trilingual children, Ares and Daphne (Photo 4.1).

Toward the end of 1973, we received an anxious phone call from Maria Tsakalakis. Paul was ill. He was being treated in Suburban Hospital, a private hospital in Bethesda, Maryland. The doctor had diagnosed lung cancer. He was admitted to the hospital with fever, coughing, and pleuritic pain, which all began suddenly. Paul lived a measured life; he had never smoked or consumed much alcohol during his life. His only excesses were a fondness for women and hard work. They asked for my help. They wanted my opinion.

That Saturday, after my morning rounds at the Veterans Administration Hospital, I went to Suburban Hospital. Paul looked completely healthy. I examined him and found no signs of anything pathological. His lab tests were normal, except for one positive cytology test of pleuritic fluids that indicated a malignancy. His doctor, however, without any confirmation of cancer through a biopsy, had begun a course of chemotherapy. That is not good medical practice. There was another patient staying in the same room with generalized metastatic cancer. I visited the pathology laboratory and verified that on the same day there had been two cytological tests of pleuritic fluids, one for Paul and one for the patient with metastatic cancer. The results of the test on the latter were reported as normal by the lab, whereas the test on Paul's pleuritic fluids showed a malignancy. This made me suspicious. It was clear that the laboratory had mixed up the results of the pleuritic fluid tests. I called in Paul's doctor and explained my concerns to him—my English was quite fluent by then— and politely suggested to him that it would be a good idea to stop chemotherapy and re-examine the patient.

Full of enthusiasm and joy because of my discovery, I was, quite innocently, most encouraging about Paul's health, both to him and Maria. I was not well acquainted with the legal system concerning malpractice in America. The minute Paul heard the good news, he got rid of all his tubes, signed a declaration in his medical record stating that he did not wish to prolong his stay or his treatment, and he went home.

Things are not always what they seem, however. One or two weeks later, we were invited to his house to celebrate the happy event. The couple's lawyer was also invited, a stout, stuffy man with an air of authority. He explained to me that in America doctors are held accountable for their mistakes, especially if the mistake is harmful rather than beneficial to the patient. I listened to him without speaking. He asked for my help. In other words, he wanted me to testify in court against Paul's physician, to present his mistakes, both diagnostic and therapeutic. He had the nerve to suggest that I would receive a 10 percent cut of whatever they were awarded from the physician's liability insurance. In addition, they would buy me a brand new Mercedes. I looked at him with scorn and disdain. The blood had risen to my head. In a firm tone of voice, I made it clear to him that I had no desire to be mixed up in any of this and continued: "If you try to involve me in your lawsuit, I'll be of no use to you because I will defend the doctor." And turning to Paul, I said to him in Greek: "I never want to see you again." I felt extremely disappointed and disgusted. They believed that I was a person with no moral values and principles, only interested in money. For the remainder of my stay in America, I never saw them again.

During the entire time I was specializing in internal medicine, I was in the habit of visiting the radiology laboratory, as well as the pathology laboratory, and studying, together with the lab specialists, the X-rays, and the pathology findings of the biopsied material taken from my patients. In that way, I formed a more complete picture of the individual I was evaluating.

One day, a professor with little interest in teaching and research was on duty at the pathology laboratory. He was having a grand old time, with his own private airplane and frequent trips to various casinos. From what I found out later, he also had a passion for playing cards. I asked him to look at the biopsies of some of my patients with me. He looked at me ironically and said to me condescendingly: "I knew that the Greeks are good cooks and that they have excellent restaurants, but I never knew they were interested in medicine." I fixed a stern gaze on him and said to him in strong language: "I'm sorry that you're treating a young colleague in this racist fashion. I demand that we look at the biopsies, and I promise you that I will make a written report about your inappropriate behavior to my superior." He became meek as a lamb. Although racism was rampant in America, but not overtly, the labels "racist" and "racism" were frightening. Needless to say, I never carried out my threat.

Starting in that academic year, I studied continuously the latest achievements in internal medicine that were published in important medical journals, such as *The New England Journal of Medicine, The Lancet,* and *Annals of Internal Medicine.* I didn't want to miss any new developments in my field. I have kept up this habit throughout my life.

It was now the spring of 1974, and I still had not decided where I would continue my training the following year. I was not too concerned, however, because I was sure that, even if I didn't get the position I wanted to begin specialization in the Department of Immunology, I would continue working within the hospital system of the Georgetown University Medical School.

One morning, after giving our report to the chairman, the chief resident informed me that Professor Hyman Zimmerman wanted me in his office that afternoon. I still remember what time of day it was. I can't describe the anxiety I went through, until it was time for our meeting. Bad thoughts ran through my head. I tried to figure out what I had done wrong. In American university hospitals, the residents' work is carefully monitored by the nurses. Every medical or behavioral error is written down and reported to the office of education. My relations with the nurses were always professional and at the same time amicable. I couldn't think of any medical errors, or inappropriate professional behavior.

At five minutes to four—throughout my life I have tried to be punctual and on time for appointments—I was in the waiting room of the chairman's office. Inside I could see Hyman, who always kept his door open, sitting at his desk shuffling through some papers (Photo 4.2). He always wore a matching jacket and bow tie, with an expensive pipe constantly in his mouth. The pleasant smell of tobacco wafted out. He could see from inside that I was waiting, and he motioned me to go into his office. He had a smile on his face, and was looking warmly at his new young colleague. "What can I offer you?" he said. "A soft drink or coffee?". His behavior relaxed me. We sat in the armchairs he had in his office. "We decided," he said to me, "to give you the position of chief resident for the educational program of internal medicine for the coming year. Your medical skills, your knowledge, and your behavior guided us in this decision." The chief resident is responsible for the education program, the working hours of the residents, and the program of rotating work shifts for the residents at the hospitals that were part of the program. In addition, he is on call twenty-four hours a day. He is the first to be notified when there is a serious administrative or medical problem in the department, or in one of the ICUs.

Feelings of joy and pride swept over me. I thanked him profusely for the honor they were bestowing on me. But without losing my composure, I immediately conveyed to him my reservations and my own wishes: "You have granted me a great honor, but at this phase of my life I do not want to be an administrator. I would very much like to find a position where I could continue my training, both at the clinical and the research levels. I want to become a clinical immunologist." He looked at me with fatherly warmth and immediately tried to satisfy my wish. What a difference between Greek and American professors. He picked up the phone and called someone named Norman. He described me to him in the most flattering terms and recommended that he hire me in his department starting on July 1, 1974. He hung up the phone and

Photo 4.2 Professor Hyman
Zimmerman

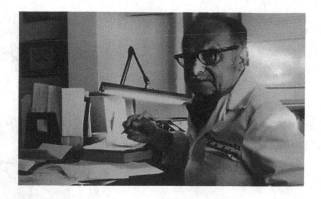

told me: "I was just speaking to Norman Talal, a famous researcher in autoimmune rheumatic diseases. He is a professor at the University of California, in San Francisco. I think that this is the ideal department for you to continue your training. During one of Norman's upcoming trips you will meet with him for an interview. He comes through Washington often. He has to see you before he can finalize his offer of a position for you." I nearly jumped for joy. At that moment, the dream motivating my emigration was finally becoming a reality.

A few weeks later, Professor Talal telephoned me. He made an appointment with me in the VIP lounge of American Airlines, at Dulles airport, at 7 p.m., on April 14. That day is still vivid in my memory. Norman, a tall, rather stout, and rugged man, was waiting in a corner of the VIP Lounge. He was unusually well dressed for an American. He looked more like a northern European professor (Photo 4.3). We discussed scientific and social issues, and he asked me about my plans for the future. From what I can tell, he was satisfied. He offered me the position of senior resident in internal medicine, with an emphasis on clinical and research studies in autoimmune rheumatic diseases. He explained to me clearly that twice a week my duties would include being in charge of night shifts as a senior resident in the internal medicine wards. One morning a week, I would be in charge of the outpatient clinic for autoimmune rheumatic disease at the Veterans Administration Hospital, and one afternoon of the outpatient clinic at the Moffitt Central University Hospital, and another morning I would be on duty at San Francisco General Hospital. The rest of the time, I would cover, as the resident in charge, all patients suspected of having autoimmune rheumatic diseases that were being treated in the internal medicine wards. "And in your free time you will have to begin your research studies," he said. I left the airport feeling elated, satisfied, and full of hope for the future.

On June 27, I packed up my Toyota Celica with all the belongings of our family, which had to be moved from Washington D.C. to San Francisco. I had studiously mapped out the states and cities I would pass through on Route 80 North. I was sure that on July 1, 1974, I would be there to take up my position, and greedily embark on the search for new knowledge and scientific conquests. Lambrini and Niki-Maria had already left for a summer vacation in Greece. On the afternoon of June 30, 1974, I was in San Francisco.

Photo 4.3 Professor
Norman Talal

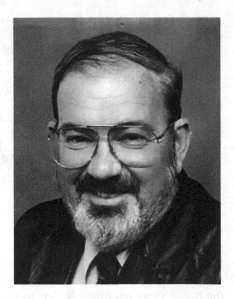

4.1.2 San Francisco

I found a room in a hotel very close to the Veterans Administration Hospital. That
was where Professor Talal's research laboratory was located. From the window of
my hotel, I could see the Pacific Ocean and the coast filled with lively, noisy seals.

Early the next morning, I was outside his office. I introduced myself to his secretary, a beautiful African-American woman, who immediately led me to his office.
The office of that great researcher was very small. It was filled with books, journals,
and notebooks. The walls were covered with diplomas and awards. "Have you had
coffee?", he asked me and offered me a cup of fragrant-smelling coffee. "Have you
found a place to live?", was his next question. "I only arrived yesterday," I answered.
"Where are you staying?" "At a hotel," I said. "Take a few days off to get yourself
settled in and then we'll talk. But before you go, come let me introduce you to my
co-workers." Don Palmer was the assistant professor. He was involved in clinical
medicine. He was not interested in laboratory research. He was responsible for the
smooth functioning of the clinical section for autoimmune rheumatic diseases. Rao
Pillarisetti, a tall, lanky, introverted Indian, was the man responsible for running
the diagnostic laboratory. I never understood exactly what his academic status was,
nor, moreover, was I interested in finding out. Ken Fye began his specialization in
autoimmune rheumatic diseases the same year as I did. The professors considered
him the best internist who had ever passed through the educational system of the California hospitals in San Francisco. The previous year he was chief resident. He was
the favorite resident of the chairman of the internal medicine department, Professor
Holly Lloyd Smith, a famous researcher in metabolic diseases.

There were many research fellows working in the laboratory: Susumi Sugai and Shigemasa Sawada from Japan; Jirayr Roubinian and Ruben Papoian, both Americans but keenly aware of their Armenian origins; Sally Davidson, with distant Irish roots; and two laboratory technicians, Edward and Ruby, two wonderful people with compassionate, sensitive personalities. They were all very friendly. They made me feel like they were pleased to have me in the section for autoimmune rheumatic diseases.

I found a large apartment, fixed it up so that it was livable and pleasant, and returned to the hospital eager to take up my post. Ken Fye and I became an inseparable scientific pair. We complemented and supplemented each other. We fired each other up with scientific questions. In no time, aside from our clinical work, we began to develop research protocols. There was still one barrier ahead of me. I believed that I now spoke and wrote excellent English. During the laboratory research meetings and bibliographical briefings, however, I thought their language was unintelligible. I gradually got up the nerve to discuss this problem with Ken. "Don't worry," he told me. It seemed that we didn't understand much because they were using technical terminology and abbreviations. For example, they referred to peripheral blood mononuclear cells as "PBMCs," and they called Concanavalin-A "Con-A," and so on and so forth. We soon found a solution. We made a list of every unknown word or abbreviation, and with the aid of medical and biological dictionaries and books we solved the puzzles. So, our adjustment to the terminology of immunology took place in a very short time.

Professors Ephraim Engelmann and Wallace Epstein were in charge of the outpatient clinic of autoimmune rheumatic diseases at the Central University Hospital. Martin Shearn was in charge of the outpatient clinic at San Francisco General Hospital. They were all serious researchers of autoimmune rheumatic diseases, and we learned important clinical lessons from those professors. They gave us the ability to diagnose and treat the most complicated and serious cases of diseases. Norman and the other professors at the Veterans Administration Hospital, including the chairman of the internal medicine department, the famous gastroenterologist Marvin Schlesinger, recognized in a short time our scholarship and talent. It was not long before they decided that we were good diagnosticians and therapists.

In my free time, when I had no clinical duties, I began experiments at the laboratory. My co-worker in these studies was Shigemasa Sawada, an unusually friendly, happy, and outgoing Japanese colleague. We communicated mostly with gestures, rather than in English. His ability to express himself in English was like mine when I first came to America. We studied the effect of thymosin, a hormone produced by the thymus gland, on T-lymphocytes, the main cells of the immune system, in patients with Sjögren's syndrome and systemic lupus erythematosus, as well as in normal controls. These diseases are known as autoimmune rheumatic diseases, because the immune system, instead of protecting the cells from foreign invaders, attacks its own cells and organs.

My collaboration with Shigemasa in the laboratory was just as productive and enjoyable as the work with Ken in the wards and outpatient clinics. We often had dinner at his house. It was a new experience for me to eat raw fish and drink sake. It tasted something like the *raki* in Ioannina, but it was much milder. After many years in San Francisco, Shigemasa eventually returned to his own country as a professor. He is a professor of rheumatology in Tokyo. Sugai, the other Japanese collaborator, was distant, and kept to himself. He kept what he was working in secret. At our research meetings, when it was his turn to present his work, it was difficult to ascertain the subject of his research. He was studying the malignant transformation of hyperactive B-lymphocytes, the cells of the immune system that produce autoantibodies, in mice with autoimmune diseases. After his training in San Francisco, he returned to Japan as a professor of immunology in Kyoto.

After the first few months adjusting to work at the university, it was clear that my income was not enough to cover the needs of my family. My self-respect, or my ego if you will, did not allow me to use money from Lambrini's family to support our family. So, after discussing the problem with Ken and with Rubinian, I got a nighttime job—"moonlighting," as it was called in American slang—once a week, usually on a weekend, at the emergency room in Kaiser Permanente Hospital. I wanted that job, because emergencies keep you alert as a clinician, and provide a respectable income.

My life as a clinician and researcher was rolling along. My successes came one after the other. Both the clinical work and the research studies produced excellent results.

Not only that, but we also had a very active social life in San Francisco. One group of friends was the Greeks. There were Professor Alexandros Kontopoulos, a famous researcher in hormonal activity of the placenta, and post-graduate students Sophia Drouva and Kostas Tsoukas. We spent unforgettable evenings together, sometimes at Kontopoulos' house and sometimes at ours. On rare occasions, we lived it up in Greek bouzouki joints. Our second group of friends consisted of my co-workers at the hospital. At our social gatherings with them there was not much food, just roasted chicken and sausages, rarely a big piece of meat, mainly salads, while the California wine flowed freely. It was also in fashion to smoke marijuana, but I didn't want to become enslaved by another bad habit. Cigarettes were enough. Our third group of friends, who happily took over the role of our parents, was the owners of our apartment, Don and Lois Wong. They often invited us to Chinatown in San Francisco and treated us to hearty meals. Don quite happily played the role of Lambrini's assistant. He ungrudgingly did our shopping along with his. He was unobtrusive, discreet, polite and, although he seemed cold, was extremely sensitive. Lois, his wife, a Japanese masseuse, generously offered her services and gave me relaxing massages when I came home tired from the hospital. She was platonically enamored of Professor Kontopoulos. She waited impatiently to be invited to our home with our Greek friends. She wanted to be in the same place as Alekos Kontopoulos. Those were the happiest times of her life.

The first six months had passed, and Norman asked me to take part, in his place, in a closed meeting of scientists in Colorado, where they would be discussing the development of a test that would contribute definitively to the diagnosis of an attack on the central nervous system by systemic lupus erythematosus. That illness is a prototype of autoimmune rheumatic disease, since it attacks all organs of the body with periodic episodes of inflammation. I accepted Norman's proposal to take part in the meeting with mixed feelings, pride on the one hand because I would be standing in for my professor, and fear, on the other, about whether I would be able to represent him scientifically. In Colorado, I found myself on a snowy mountain in Colorado Springs, in an excellent hotel. At that meeting, all the big names in the study of autoimmune rheumatic diseases participated: Morris Ziff, Eng Tan, Roger Williams, dressed as always like a Texas cowboy, and Mary Betty Stevens from Johns Hopkins.

The meeting began. They were all ten or twenty years older than me, except for one other participant who looked very young. He spoke English with a Spanish accent. "He must be a colleague of Donato Alarcón-Segovia," I thought. "He probably sent him as a stand-in, like Talal sent me." But I quickly realized I had made a mistake. He himself was Alarcón-Segovia. Alarcón-Segovia, when I was just beginning my specialization, had already published many important clinical and research papers on practically every autoimmune rheumatic disease. During that meeting we became friends. When, many years later, he found out that I was returning to Greece as a professor of medicine, he came over to me at a conference and said to me: "Haralampe,"—he was the only person in America who didn't call me Harry—"Your country is just like mine. Don't listen to anyone, do whatever you think you should." How many times have I remembered the advice he gave me. I took his advice and have never gone wrong.

My mentor Norman Talal was an accomplished scholar on immunology and the pathogenesis of autoimmune diseases, but completely indifferent to clinical medicine. Once a week, he carried out the director's rounds to patients. Each patient's data gave him the opportunity to teach immunology. He used patients' data as a springboard to analyze pathogenetic mechanisms of disease. If the patient was suffering from nephritis, for example, he would teach us how the complexes of autoantigens and autoantibodies activate a series of immune-proteins in the blood, which are called complement proteins, and how the activation of these proteins fuels inflammation and leads to damage in tissues and organs. The physiology and the pathology of complement proteins is one of the more difficult areas of immunology. He taught it very digestibly. So, his way of teaching saved you many hours of studying in order to understand difficult medical concepts. He was prone to irony and frowned on discussions about which immunosuppressive medicines and in what dosage to prescribe for a patient. For Norman these were superfluous details. On the other hand, he would become ecstatic with the results of experiments. As soon as he got the results, he had the unique ability to synthesize them and develop a theory. He was exceptionally friendly with colleagues who contributed to his research, and completely indifferent to anyone unproductive.

In my earlier description of my colleagues, I neglected to mention Jean Louis Feldmann, a Frenchman, who had just finished his specialization in rheumatology and had come to Norman's lab as a research fellow in immunology. After more than a year of very hard work in the laboratory, Jean Louis managed to complete a study on the subpopulation of lymphocytes called K-lymphocytes (K standing for "killer") in the blood sera of patients with autoimmune rheumatic disease. That study was accepted by the *Journal of Clinical Investigation.* The journal accepts important experimental studies from all branches of internal medicine.

As for Norman, aside from the prescribed weekly research meetings, one could also meet with him alone, one-on-one. These meetings always happened outside of the laboratory. He liked having a discussion either while walking along the endless garden of the hospital, which looked out on the Pacific Ocean, or while having a midday meal. During these meetings, he didn't make suggestions about experiments, but rather wanted to draw you out to gauge the depth and breadth of your thinking on research. He used Socratic dialogue. For example, he would ask: "What is the dominant inflammatory cell in the tissues affected by myositis, that is, inflammation of the muscles?". He would listen to the answer and continue with another question: "How does that cell cause the damage in the myocytes?". He always wanted the answer to be well documented. After you answered, he would continue: "What experiment supports your viewpoint?". "Did you analyze the experiment?". "If you were doing that experiment, what would you have done differently?". "What is the bibliographical source that shows that lymphotoxin, a substance that is produced by activated T-lymphocytes, caused the muscular damage?". "Where did you find it?". If he disagreed, he did not say so in words. You would see it in the expression on his face. Those discussions not only boosted your self-confidence, because you knew the mechanisms of those diseases, but they made you aware of scientific data that you had not thought about, or had not taken seriously. Without your even trying, they increased your capacity to formulate scientific questions. They stimulated your imagination.

Extremely pleased with my experiments and their results, I thought it might be a good idea to do some basic studies in immunology, by enrolling in a Ph.D. program at the University of California, in Berkeley. I talked this over with my professor. He soon convinced me—I still don't know if I did the right thing by listening to him—that it would be a waste of time. "In the five years it will take you to get your Ph.D. you will have become a well-known researcher," he said. So my plan ended unsuccessfully.

The Talals had a fantastic house in Tiburon, a very expensive area across from San Francisco. Whenever he had a visiting professor there, he would invite his whole department to his house, from the secretary and technicians to the scientific personnel (Photo 4.4). He greatly enjoyed arranging these social events, and we enjoyed attending them. Aside from his scientific interests, Norman was a gourmand and a passionate collector of such things as Coca Cola trays and matchboxes in every size, shape, and color.

Our research was proceeding quickly. The results were accepted at the annual conference of clinical research. It took place every year in Atlantic City, a seaside resort town in New Jersey. I was the only co-worker that Talal took with him, as my research had been accepted for oral presentation at the conference. We arrived there on Holy Saturday. Our paper entitled "In vitro effect of thymosin on T-lymphocyte rosette formation in rheumatic diseases" was scheduled to be presented on Easter Sunday at 9 a.m. To save money, we shared a room in the hotel. After dropping off our luggage, we each went our own way. I went to follow the afternoon session, whose subject was clinical immunology. I listened with great interest to the papers presented there. I took notes. I made plans for future studies. Suddenly, I saw three

Photo 4.4 Author, Norman Talal, Shigemasa Sawada and Susumi Sugai at Talal's house

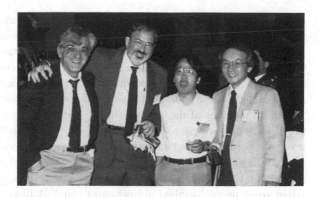

familiar faces next to me. After some hesitation, I recognized them: Nikos Madias, Philippos Tsihlis, and Apostolos Vagenakis. The first two had been classmates of mine, both excellent students. We went abroad the same year. Nikos was a specialist in nephrology and Philippos in hematology. Nikos Madias, after many years of study and a significant scientific output, is today a professor of nephrology and the chairman of the internal medicine department at Tufts University Medical Center, in Boston.

Apostolos, who was seven years older than us, was already an internationally recognized researcher in endocrinology, and a professor at Boston University Medical School. He was elected professor the same time as me and was chairman of the internal medicine department at the University of Patras Medical School. He created an exemplary internal medicine department, with all the specialties. He produced excellent physicians. He was a shining example of a person combining all the qualities of an educator, clinician, and researcher. He retired several years ago.

There we were, three friends from Greece in the same hall, at the same conference. We went outside so we could talk more easily. Our excitement and surprise cannot be described on a mere piece of paper. At once, we decided to go out to a nightclub with Greek music. We ate, we drank, we danced, and many hours after midnight we decided to go back to our hotels. When I arrived at my room in the hotel, I saw through a crack that the light was on. I snuck in guiltily and found Norman standing there, waiting anxiously for me. "Where were you?", he asked angrily. "It's Holy Saturday," I told him "and I went to church with some friends." "I never knew that a Greek-Orthodox Church is a place to get drunk," he said, and in a very severe and angry tone of voice, he insisted I take a cold shower. After my shower, there was yet another damper in store for me. He obliged me to practice several times the paper I was going to present at 9 a.m. the next morning. If I remember correctly, I hardly slept that night. But we had earned our outing. My evening with the Greeks was worth that trouble and more.

At the end of each academic year, in June, Norman took everyone in his department for a long weekend, from Thursday afternoon to Sunday evening, to Yosemite National Park, an idyllic spot in California. Every morning, for two or three hours, we had a review of new scientific data on immunology and autoimmune diseases, called a bibliographical briefing in medical language, and after that we were free to go hiking, riding, or engage in other activities, amid amazing natural beauty.

In July of 1975, I had completed my three years of training in internal medicine. I took the examinations of the American College of Physicians. They were complicated and long. Even though the percentage of successful candidates was only 25%, the notice had my name among those who passed. I was now an internist with a capital "I" and a member of the college. In my second academic year in San Francisco, my clinical duties were reduced to one-third. Two younger colleagues took over the positions of resident, and we had a lot more time for experiments in the laboratory. In the fall, Ken and I were assigned to write two chapters of the book *Clinical and Basic Immunology* for Lange Publications. Everything was going extraordinarily well, when some news disturbed my peace of mind. Although Professor Talal, because of our excellent performance, had promised Ken and me that we would become assistant professors starting in July 1976, the decision taken by the university was different. Ken was promoted, while I stayed behind, if I wished, as a fellow in the department for a third year. I did not answer this proposal. I thought it would not be useful to spend a third year in the same department, nor would it be useful for my future scientific career. I felt a need to familiarize myself with the thinking and the experiments of other researchers. I thought that this latest development was unfair to me. I was angry, but I kept my anger under control. I didn't show it. However, I soon found an opportunity to leave San Francisco. Professor Talal tried to dissuade me, to no avail. I can understand why he was not pleased with my decision.

In spite of all this, I decided to go someplace familiar, and where else but the Washington D.C. area? From the time that I was in training at the affiliated hospitals of Georgetown University Medical School, I had a secret wish to one day work at the National Institutes of Health (NIH). I left San Francisco with my mentor, Yiannis Papavassileiou, who was visiting and staying with me at the time. We stayed at a hotel called the Ramada Inn, next to the NIH.

In the morning, I went out looking for work. I soon found myself in the office of the director of the branch of arthritic and rheumatic disorders at the National Institute of Arthritic and Metabolic Disease. I asked for an appointment, and fortunately the secretaries made me an appointment with John L. Decker at twelve noon on the same day (Photo 4.5). It was December, it was cold, raining lightly and the wind could whisk you away like dried leaves. I had Professor Papavassileiou with me. I left him in the library of the NIH. When I met with Dr. Decker, I gave him my curriculum vitae and I asked him if it was possible to find me a job. He was tall and polite and not very talkative. During my interview, he telephoned Norman. From what I could tell, Norman described me in the most positive terms. He asked Decker, however, to persuade me to return to San Francisco.

After the information he got from Norman about my progress in San Francisco, Decker telephoned various section heads, and eventually he found an available position for me. It was in the laboratory of Thomas Chused, on the second floor of the building. Chused and I had something in common. He had also been Talal's student.

Despite my unexpected departure from San Francisco, Professor Talal and I maintained a lively, dynamic, and productive scientific relationship. At the scientific

Photo 4.5 Dr. John L. Decker

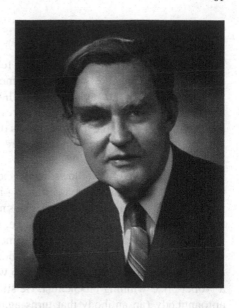

conferences in our field, we always found the time to meet. We would continue our Socratic dialogues. We would pose questions to each other, and stimulate one another to be scientifically creative. I will never forget a discussion we had that discouraged me from doing an important experiment. Even though many years have passed, it seems like that discussion took place yesterday. I asked him why he believed that "in the laboratory the red blood cells of a sheep attach themselves to human T-lymphocytes and rosettes are formed." He couldn't give me a satisfactory answer. I told him enthusiastically that I would study that phenomenon. He found a thousand reasons why I shouldn't. In the end, he convinced me. Several years later, the phenomenon was studied at length by others. Their research led to the discovery of adhesion molecules. These molecules are important in the movement of leukocytes and their adhesion to the damaged area.

Norman came to see us many times in Ioannina as a visiting professor, and I made similar visits to him in Dallas, Texas, where he had moved from San Francisco and was serving as director of the section on autoimmune rheumatic diseases. We wrote scientific papers together, and many of my students did graduate research work in his laboratory. We authored a book together on Sjögren's syndrome that is considered a classic. It has now been several years, however, since the scientific output of this important scholar of immunology ceased completely. He contracted a serious illness that inhibited his ability to speak and cut off his communication with the rest of the world. My loss of communication with Norman was very painful and sad and it cost me dearly.

My last visit to New York in the early 1990s was a very somber occasion. No longer was he the sharp-witted, incisively thoughtful researcher I had once known and admired. Only the shell of his body remained.

4.1.3   Back to Washington, D.C.

In January 1976, I was hired as a research fellow at Tom Chused's laboratory. Tom was studying the pathogenesis of autoimmune rheumatic diseases, using New Zealand mice as an experimental animal model. Those mice, and in particular the hybrid of the first generation of white mice, which were crossed with black mice, were predisposed to developing, within the first six months of their life, systemic lupus erythematosus, which clinically and immunologically resembles systemic lupus erythematosus in humans.

There were two other fellows in that section: Stuart Kassan and Masashi Akizuki (Photo 4.6). Stuart had done his training in internal medicine at the George Washington University Medical Center. He was not interested in experiments; he was a clinical researcher, friendly, polite, talkative, from a well-to-do family, always dressed in brand-name clothes. He quickly became my friend. Azikuki was a rheumatologist from Tokyo. He only worked in the laboratory. He was well dressed, introverted, reserved, and almost anti-social. He too was from a good family, the son-in-law of a Nobel-prize-winning biochemist. He still believed that he had discovered another autoantibody (an antibody that turns against autoantigens). He named it anti-Ha. Unfortunately, he had simply reinvented the wheel. That autoantibody had been described by three other research teams before him: Jones, in the late 1950s, had named it anti-SjD; Morris Reichlin, in the late 1970s, had named it anti-La, and Eng Tan, in the mid-1970s, had called it anti-SSB. Azikuki never discussed what experiment he was working on or what results he had. Everything was a state secret.

I rented a large apartment in Wheaton, Maryland. I had let Lambrini know that our new place of residence was Washington D.C. She was in Athens with Niki-Maria, so that she could take her bar exams. She was pleased with my decision. Washington was closer to Athens. I threw myself into my work. Soon, I was doing surgery on mice. I acquired the ability to remove the spleen, or the thymus gland from mice. Soon the experiments paid off. We showed that the B-lymphocytes of the mice, which are prone to spontaneously developing lupus in their sixth month of life, were activated from the very first week of their life. That study was published in the *Journal of Immunology*.

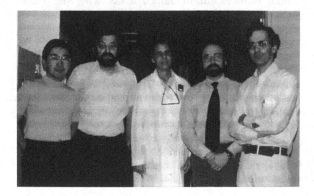

Photo 4.6 From left to right: Masashi Akizuki, author, Eleonora, Stuart Kassan and Tom Chused

We soon completed experiments that studied the condition of the T-cells and the macrophages of those mice. Before we submitted those studies for publication, and after many corrections, we would give the paper to Chused for his approval. Another comrade and tireless researcher on all those experiments was Marilyn Boehm-Truitt, a basic researcher in immunochemistry, the wife of the chairman of the biochemistry department of the George Washington University Medical School. Aside from the hard work, on many afternoons, Marilyn and I would go to a private airport, in Fredrickson, for pilot training flights. After a few months, I gave up that hobby. It was time-consuming and expensive. In all the experiments, I also had the valuable help of Eleonora, a technician in Tom Chused's group. A middle-aged biracial woman, quiet and hard-working, she knew our experiments through and through. She had no family responsibilities. She was at the laboratory from dawn to dusk. The department secretary was Doris Light, a short, chubby woman with little inclination for work. She became almost hostile whenever someone gave her a new paper to type.

At this point it might be expedient and useful, especially for my younger colleagues, to mention two more educational procedures. First, let me outline the arduous process that every research or clinical study had to go through back then, before it was submitted to a biomedical journal for publication. When all the experimental or clinical data had been collected and analyzed and the text of the study was in its final form, the institute required that the study be evaluated by two independent researchers from the institute, who were not part of the research team that had done the study. The evaluators did a scrupulous examination of the study, with written comments, corrections, and clarifications, and they often asked for additional experiments before giving their approval. Upon completion of the internal evaluation, the final review of the study was performed by the director of the institute, or the associate director. These internal reviews provided important scientific benefits to the researchers and contributed substantially to optimizing and improving the research study to be published. The groundbreaking information in the papers that were put out by the NIH and the thorough review of the papers, before they were submitted for publication, led to the acceptance of most of the papers by the best-known scientific biomedical journals.

The second educational process was meant to develop young researchers' skills in teaching and speaking. A researcher who had to present his or her work at a conference had to first present it two or three times at a meeting of the whole section. The point of this procedure was to improve the quality of slides, present one's research more analytically, and discuss one's results as fully and clearly as possible. This explains why researchers, who are trained in this kind of procedure, are meticulous analysts and excellent teachers of medicine.

My involvement in experimental immunology soon uncovered my deficiencies in the basic sciences. In Greece, during my years as a student, we were never taught current biochemistry, molecular biology, basic immunology, or statistics.

To correct these deficiencies, I enrolled in post-graduate studies at the NIH. Through the courses I took, I became familiar with the fundamental rules that govern the functioning of living organisms. The courses in statistics enhanced my ability to better organize clinical studies and evaluate the importance of the results.

Aside from the experiments and the nighttime graduate studies, I also had clinical obligations. One morning a week, from eight to one, I worked in the outpatient clinic for autoimmune rheumatic diseases. We examined patients who had been referred to our department by doctors all over America. This was yet another important lesson to round out the knowledge I acquired studying autoimmune rheumatic diseases. When office hours were over, for two hours we gathered in the classroom, and with John L. Decker coordinating us, we discussed cases with especially difficult diagnostic or therapeutic problems. There, I came into contact with the sharpest minds of physicians, teachers, and researchers.

The researchers in our department, all with very strong personalities, worked beautifully together, thanks to the amiable but austere personality of Dr. Decker. He was fully aware at every moment of what each of the members of his department was doing on a clinical, research, and personal level. He knew details about the illness and the progress of all the patients being followed by our department. The notes he took during all our meetings were very helpful in this regard. That distinguished educator was not only an excellent physician and researcher; he also had great sensitivity and a gentle way of interacting with the patients being treated. He was quite tall. His appearance was awe-inspiring. I believe he knew this, and because of this he would kneel when examining his patients to make them feel more comfortable. He did not want to tower over them because of his height.

Still ingrained in my memory is the sharp, discerning, imaginative, and unfailingly knowledgeable mind of Dr. Alfred (Fred) D. Steinberg (Photo 4.7). Fred and I did important experiments together. We crossbred mice from New Zealand with a tendency to develop lupus with mice whose B-lymphocytes were not functioning. The hybrid mice were cured of the disease. That study showed the important contribution of B-lymphocytes, the cells of the immune system that produce antibodies, to understanding the pathogenesis of systemic lupus erythematosus. Many years later, these findings were put to use by the pharmaceutical industry. Today, the elimination of B-lymphocytes from peripheral blood is used as a therapy for patients with systemic lupus erythematosus and other autoimmune diseases. Steinberg's scientific talents were supplemented by his intellectual depth, thoroughness, and in some cases, the ability to make quick decisions, a quality shared by Dr. Paul Plotz, another distinguished member of our branch. Dr. Chused only sporadically attended the clinical seminars, with no substantial input. Patients were a chore for him. He was shy and remote, and he delighted in working for hours on the cellular analyzer and separator, an electronic machine whose function is based on laser beams. He was not a physician by nature. Another abundant source of learning was our Friday morning meetings. We would study, under a multi-headed microscope, the kidney biopsies of patients with autoimmune rheumatic diseases. This scientific procedure was coordinated by the nephrologist and researcher Jim Balow. The NIH was an amazing place for learning, with a wealth of knowledge. It gave physicians an opportunity to stimulate their imagination and bolster their expertise.

Researchers were not the only purveyors of knowledge working at the NIH. That research center attracted as speakers the best-known clinical and basic researchers involved in the creation of new biomedical knowledge. Many of them had been

Photo 4.7 Dr. Alfred D. Steinberg and wife Suzan with author and Alice Smolen

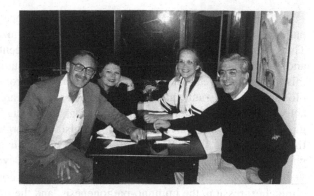

awarded the Nobel Prize. Every Monday morning, when the so-called "yellow page" was circulated, that is, the program of the Institute's scientific events, you didn't know which talk or lecture to attend. One was better than the other.

Among the more memorable talks, to name just a few, were those by C. M. Edelman and R. R. Porter on the chemical structure of antibodies, by Carleton Gajdusek on new mechanisms for contracting and transmitting infectious diseases, and by B. Benacerraf on genetically determined structures on the surface of cells that regulate immunological reactions, that is, histocompatibility antigens.

Training, clinical work, and research at the NIH required more than twelve hours a day. Our interest in learning mitigated our physical tiredness. I never left work feeling exhausted. I returned home late at night impatient for the night to end, so that I could be at the laboratory early in the morning to continue my experiments and further improve my clinical and experimental medical skills.

In addition to studying the functional state of immunological cells of mice with systemic lupus erythematosus, we tried to determine the cause of the activation of the immune system. We studied whether those mice had been infected by onco- genic, ecotrophic, slow viruses, meaning viruses that the mice host in their bodies that very gradually become infectious. Those experiments were conducted with the help of another researcher, Dr. Sandy Morse. We did thousands of experiments, and put in endless hours of work, all with no results. But the experience I gained was unparalleled and has stayed with me.

The days were going by and Dr. Chused had not commented on the other two experimental studies we had submitted to him. They were buried in his desk drawer. I tried many times to ascertain what he planned to do with those studies, but I never got an answer. My questions were answered late that spring. Those studies had been presented at a conference on basic science, held in Cold Spring Harbor, in Long Island, New York. In the book of the proceedings of the conference they were given a prominent place, with one slight difference: my name was second, after Tom's name. I swallowed my anger and my disappointment. I understood from Tom's behavior that he didn't want me to continue my experiments on mice. I had to find something else to work on.

In San Francisco, I had acquired a lot of experience with Sjögren's syndrome patients. Professor Talal was an internationally recognized expert on this disease. The syndrome occurs frequently. It affects about 1 percent of the female population, and it is the most classic prototype for the study of autoimmune diseases. Why is this happening? Because the individuals who suffer from this disease have in their bloodstream many autoantibodies, and the tissues that are affected are infiltrated by activated lymphocytes. The main organs that are affected are not only the exocrine glands (the tear and salivary glands), but also other organs, such as the lungs, the liver, the kidneys, the muscles, and the blood vessels. In a great proportion of these patients, the disease develops into a malignancy of B-lymphocytes (lymphoma). I visited Dr. Decker and informed him that I wanted to concentrate my study on the clinical expression, the immuno-pathogenesis, and the treatment of this syndrome. I found him in agreement and most amenable to this idea. Tom was in charge of research on this syndrome, but he was not interested in human disease. Stuart was the one who did clinical studies on that syndrome. I helped him finish a study that described the relative danger for patients with Sjögren's syndrome of developing lymphomas and the association of class-II histocompatibility antigens with those patients. The immunogenetic research was planned, carried out, and written up by Stuart. All that day, Tom was busy with various other things. He invited us to his house, one Sunday morning, to give us his corrections and comments on the text of our study. At 11 o'clock in the morning we knocked on the gate of his house, which was in an expensive neighborhood called Chevy Chase, located on the border of northwest Washington D.C. and Maryland.

He greeted us in the sitting room. We sat down on a sofa, and without wasting any words, he began giving us his suggestions concerning our study.

His wife, a psychiatrist, was busy preparing something in the kitchen. With a total lack of respect for the rules of proper etiquette, she complained to her husband that she didn't want him to work on Sundays, or bring colleagues to the house. Tom paid no attention to her grumbling. That made her furious. She came over to us holding the cake she was making. For a moment I thought she was going to offer us a piece. But the cake was meant for someone else. Howling, she brought it down on Tom's head like a hat. All we got were a few stray bits. We had no choice but to abandon that "hospitable" house.

The following day, we continued our scientific discussion in the laboratory. Even though Stuart had done all the work, Dr. Chused insisted that his name appear first on the published study. A quarrel of epic proportions ensued, but in the end, his point of view was upheld. "The chief is always right," as the famous medical teacher David R. Hawkins was fond of saying.

Stuart and I remained friends and continued working together. I visited him in Colorado and he visited us in Greece often, sometimes for vacation and sometimes to take part in international conferences we organized. We have authored scientific articles and reviews for medical journals and books together. After studying the records of our patients, we described the clinical and immunological differences in individuals suffering from the syndrome itself and patients suffering from rheumatoid arthritis, who simultaneously exhibit symptoms of Sjögren's syndrome. In those studies, we proposed that Sjögren's syndrome be called primary, when patients do not exhibit clinical or immunological manifestations of another autoimmune rheumatic disease, and secondary, when the syndrome manifests itself in patients with rheumatoid arthritis. In collaboration with Dean Mann, an immunogeneticist, we showed the genetic differences between these two groups of patients. Our studies were published in the most prominent medical journals. In this way, I found my own way and in essence became independent of Tom's administrative oversight. My independence from him did me a lot of good. It helped me to mature, and it allowed me to think up my own scientific subjects and organize my own experiments. I did not stop admiring him as a person, however. I never forgot that during a difficult time in my life he accepted me in his section. I always put his name in my publications, but second to last. Last was always Dr. Decker.

Our social life in Washington was more extensive than in San Francisco. My colleague from Providence Hospital, Tryphon Vlagopoulos, and his family lived in the same apartment complex. When I started my specialization in America, Tryphon was the chief resident in the Department of Internal Medicine. He was a well-read physician, a courteous man with a low-key personality. His greatest weakness was Marika, his wife and sole companion throughout his life. We went through thick and thin together. In 1976, they lost their daughter to leukemia. We were the godparents of their second child, Panayotis. In early 1976, they had also returned to Washington, but from Nebraska, where Tryphon had been trained as an allergist. On Sundays, when I was not working, we spent the day at the home of Peter Protos, the gynecologist. His house was open to all Greeks, whether diplomats, military attachés, or scientists. You could find the entire Greek community of Washington there. You could hear all the news from Greece, and indulge yourselves by eating exceptional food, everything from Argentinian steaks to Maryland crabs and New England lobsters. You could have anything that struck your fancy. Very often, we were invited to the homes of colleagues from our department. Drs. Steinberg and Plotz were particularly hospitable. You could meet very interesting people in their homes: poets, authors, journalists, and lawyers.

Come spring, Lambrini and I had completed the necessary time to apply to change our visas from educational to immigrant. We were eligible for the so-called green card. Our experience with the immigration service was disappointing. People were pushed into lines like animals waiting to be corralled. The employees were demeaning and racist in attitude. In recent years, this picture often comes into my mind when I see long queues of immigrants pushing and shoving each other in front of the police station on Alexandras Avenue, in Ambelokipoi, waiting to get their much-sought-after immigration papers. We were patient. We finally got our green cards. With this card, I could now get a better position at the NIH.

In June of 1976, I took exams at the American College of Rheumatology to be certified as a rheumatologist, and I passed. The title of rheumatologist, however, was not enough for me. It held me back and limited me. I was an internal medicine physician, with a specialization in autoimmune rheumatic diseases. I wanted my specialty to reflect a broader range of my scientific capabilities and thinking. There were

Photo 4.8 Author, Drs.
Abner Notkins and Francis
McCartney

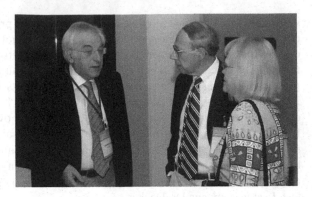

no examinations to acquire, on paper at least, the title of specialist in autoimmune rheumatic diseases.

The next academic year was very productive. My clinical duties continued, and my research collaborations increased. Together with a team headed by Dr. Abner Notkins (Photo 4.8), we discovered that interferon, an antiviral protein, was circulating in the blood of patients with active systemic lupus erythematosus and Sjögren's syndrome. This discovery indirectly indicated that in the pathogenesis of those diseases an important role is most likely played by viral infections. That study was accepted for presentation at the plenary session of the annual scientific meeting on immunology in Atlantic City, New Jersey. I presented the study there, and it was subsequently published in *The New England Journal of Medicine*.

With the team of Steve Katz, and in particular his colleague Tom Lowley, who was later appointed dean of the medical school in Atlanta, Georgia, we studied the immune-complexes in the blood of patients with Sjögren's syndrome, as well as the function of cells of the reticuloendothelial system. In addition to the scientific work at the NIH, every Saturday or Sunday, I worked for twelve hours at the emergency room of the General Hospital in southeast Washington, an especially dangerous area. It was a poor, African-American neighborhood. Many of the men were out of work, and alcoholics or drug addicts. The women were typically unmarried, with many children, and living on welfare. The emergency room at the hospital treated all kinds of patients and illnesses: alcoholics with symptoms in every system of the body: the central nervous system, the liver, the pancreas, the gastrointestinal, and hematopoietic systems; acute or chronic infections in undernourished individuals and drug addicts; myocardial infarctions, congestive heart failure, wounds from firearms or knives. It was an incredible experience. I worked in that hospital during the entire time we lived in Washington.

Many nights in the emergency room, Tryphon Vlagopoulos worked there with me. We supplemented each other in our physical, mental, and medical abilities. Although Tryphon was an excellent physician, he often avoided cases that required quick therapeutic decisions. I filled in for him in that regard. On the other hand, Tryphon was ideal for patients who needed more conversation than action. In the same hospital, in the Department of Radiology, an outgoing, friendly technician named Roula Doukata was working. She always had a smile on her face. Many nights after work, we had breakfast at dawn at some all-night restaurant. Several years later, Roula and her childhood sweetheart Dr. Marinos Dalakas joined their lives together in marriage.

One night, while returning home from the hospital after my shift, I noticed an illuminated house with a sign announcing that the tenant was a famous palm reader. Without delay I parked the car and went inside to meet her. She was a middle-aged Indian lady. After studying my palm, she predicted all the important events in my life, everything from illnesses and family matters to professional accomplishments. And as each of the predicted events came to pass, I remembered that lady.

Toward the end of spring, 1977, I received two excellent pieces of news. The Georgetown University Medical School awarded me the title of clinical assistant professor of internal medicine. That title entailed important obligations: I had to work as an attending physician in charge of a working group that consisted of a second-year resident, two first-year interns, and four final-year medical students. That obligation was for two months a year at the Central University Hospital, and two months at the Veterans Administration Hospital. I was in the clouds. "This honorary position," I said to myself, "is an opportunity to keep myself up-to-date in internal medicine."

The second honor came with recognition by the NIH of my progress as a clinician and a researcher. Tom was moved from his position as the chief of research on Sjögren's syndrome to the department where the complicated machine was located, the one that separated and analyzed blood cells, and I formally took over his section. The section had two positions for research fellows. Eleonora and Doris both stayed with me. The funding for our research was considerable.

Lambrini, after taking a wide range of courses in law school, also found her way. She enrolled as a graduate student in a Ph.D. program at the Hastings Center in the Kennedy Institute of Ethics, with a major in bioethics. So, everyone was now happy.

4.2 Teacher and Researcher

Starting in July 1977, I left the secure position of research fellow and assumed a leadership post: chief of research on Sjögren's syndrome. This was not only quite an honor, but also a tremendous responsibility. I had to prove that I was up to the job. In developed countries, you are under constant surveillance. It is not like in Greece, where once you become a professor you no longer need to do anything. No one checks your performance. No one evaluates you.

My first two fellows were the Canadian rheumatologist Dr. Jack Karsh and the American Dr. Neil Stahl, both excellent physicians, but uninterested in laboratory research. I assigned Jack Karsh two studies: one on thyroid gland disease in patients with Sjögren's syndrome and one on their ability to mount an immune response to the pneumococcal vaccine. He was thorough and hard-working. In the two years we worked together, he completed both studies. They were published in *Arthritis and*

Rheumatism. He eventually became a professor of rheumatology in Canada. Neil took part in some of the branch studies. I still see him often. He is a rheumatologist in Washington, D.C. He is always friendly, and always has a good word for me and my scientific contribution to his development as a physician.

My new academic positions increased my clinical obligations. Three months a year, I was the attending physician for the patients in the arthritis and rheumatism ward on the ninth floor of the NIH clinical center. I supervised the work of two fellows in rheumatology training. I was their teacher. This commitment was in addition to my duties at the outpatient clinic at the NIH and my clinical and teaching responsibilities at Georgetown University Medical School. These were not chores for me, they were all a pleasure. My clinical responsibilities enhanced my skills. This was, moreover, what I had always wanted: to be a clinician, a teacher, and a researcher.

Together with the oncology team of the National Cancer Institute, and in particular with the hematologist Dr. Allan Gratwohl, we studied patients who had undergone allogenic bone marrow transplants, that is, they had been implanted with the bone marrow of another unrelated individual. One complication from these transplants was the appearance of a chronic reaction of the transplanted immune cells of the bone marrow against the cells and organs of the host, that is, the individual who received the bone marrow. We showed that this condition, which caused chronic activation of T-lymphocytes, led to the development of autoimmune diseases, such as Sjögren's syndrome, scleroderma, lupus, and biliary cirrhosis. Alan and I worked harmoniously and pleasantly together. We considered our participation to be equal. And so, we decided to leave whose name would be first on our papers to chance. We tossed a coin and Alan won. The papers were published in the *Annals of Internal Medicine.* I presented the results of our study at the plenary session of the annual conference, in Atlantic City. Alan is now a professor of hematology in Switzerland, and has contributed significantly to that specialty of medicine.

In collaboration with Anthony Fauci (Photo 4.9), director of the Institute of Allergic and Infectious Diseases, we studied the activation status of lymphocytes in the peripheral blood and bone marrow of patients with autoimmune diseases. One paper was published in the *Journal of Clinical Investigation* and the other in *Arthritis and Rheumatism.* This was yet another feather in my research and clinical cap. Fauci was an exceptional researcher at every stage of his training. He was extraordinarily intelligent, a workaholic—there was no relaxing on weekends for him—with an incomparable medical imagination. He was athletic; he would run five miles every morning before he started work. He was for me the most shining example of a conscientious researcher. Throughout my medical career, he has been my prototype.

My experience teaching, both at the Georgetown University Medical School and at the institute, was the cornerstone of my overall development as a teacher of medicine. The residents at both medical centers were excellently prepared for the medical cases they were responsible for. They did their reading and prepared questions regarding the further diagnostic and therapeutic treatment of their patients. I owe a lot to that teaching experience.

Photo 4.9 Dr. Anthony
Fauci

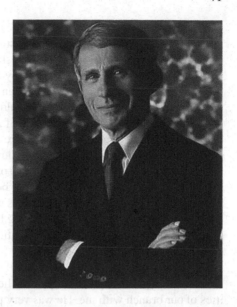

To improve my clinical skills, I attended two more functions at the NIH. Every Wednesday, I did my best to be present at Fauci's educational rounds for his institute's patients. There, I had the opportunity to encounter all kinds of patients, with systemic vasculitis. These disorders were Fauci's passion. He was the person who developed the therapy for them. Vasculitis had become a focus of interest for me during my time in San Francisco.

Every Thursday morning, dermatologists from the Washington area would bring difficult dermatological cases for discussion. At these discussions, I perfected my skills in diagnosing skin rashes. The skin is one of the organs that is attacked by autoimmune diseases. It is imperative for any physician treating these diseases to be familiar with their dermatologic manifestations. I am grateful to Steve Katz for his help in consolidating my medical knowledge.

The critiques from the Georgetown Hospital residents I was teaching were positive. Every year during evaluation I received excellent comments. That led the Georgetown University Medical School, after two years, to promote me to the rank of clinical associate professor of internal medicine.

The time I could spend with my family on excursions and on cultivating the mind and spirit was very limited. During all my years in America, especially the last four years, enjoying ourselves in this way was a rare occasion. Only very infrequently did we attend a concert of Greek or foreign music at the John F. Kennedy Center for the Performing Arts. On the odd Sunday, we would go to an art exhibition at the Torpedo Factory Art Center in Alexandria, Virginia. It had been converted into an exhibition hall for young artists. These limited occasions, which were supplemented over time by visits to art galleries in cities I was visiting for professional reasons, awoke in me a taste for learning about art.

Excursions outside of our area were few and far between and, with one exception, not longer than a day. Our favorite destinations were Annapolis, a lovely seaside town in Maryland, and Colonial Williamsburg, the old capital of the state of Virginia, which was reconstructed in the 1950s by John D. Rockefeller; and also, downtown Washington D.C., to visit monuments and museums. The only trip we made on a weekend was to Florida, so the kids could visit Disneyland.

In the summer of 1977, a classmate of mine from Greece, Dimitris Goules, came to Washington. He wanted to learn more about autoimmune rheumatic diseases. It was also a long-time wish of his to write a doctoral thesis. He was specializing in rheumatology at the Evangelismos Hospital, in Athens, under the supervision of Dr. Giorgos Fostiropoulos. Giorgos had been trained in Boston, and he had few but important studies to his name; the studies were on the role of complement proteins in autoimmune rheumatic diseases. During his student years at the Athens University Medical School, Dimitris was conscientious in his studies and a good student. He came from Astakos, Aitolia-Acarnania.

My apartment was empty. The family was on vacation in Greece. So, to help reduce his expenses, I put him up at my house. He attentively followed all the activities of our branch with me. He was very preoccupied with scientific issues. He had thousands of questions, but he could often be tiring. He wanted to improve himself. It was not too long until he confessed another wish to me. He asked me discreetly if I could assign him a clinical project for his doctoral thesis. At that time, I had decided to gather clinical, laboratory, and histopathological data from the records of patients with systemic scleroderma and eosinophilic fasciitis. I wanted to figure out the similarities and differences between those two diseases. Scleroderma is a chronic condition characterized by excessive deposits of collagen, a basic protein, in the skin, the lungs, and the digestive system. Eosinophilic fasciitis was recently described by Professor Lawrence Schulman at the Johns Hopkins University Medical School. This disease, which today is known as Schulman's syndrome, is characterized by inflammation and swelling of the fascia (the fibrous tissue that separates the skin from the muscles) and mainly attacks the limbs. Schulman had transferred out of Johns Hopkins and was working as scientific director at the National Institute of Arthritis and Musculoskeletal and Skin Disease. He was in charge of distributing, after stringent evaluation, funds from the institute to various medical schools throughout the country. I put Dimitris to work. He very quickly collected the data I had asked him for. Dimitris' collection of scientific data on that disease earned him a doctoral degree. With the data we had gathered, we wrote an article presenting the clinical, laboratory, and histological similarities and differences between Schulman's syndrome and scleroderma.

I submitted the article to two researchers at the institute who had not been involved in the study. I received positive comments. I gave the article and the positive comments to Dr. Schulman to get his approval. Days went by and I had no response. I didn't want to go through what I did with Dr. Chused again. I asked Dr. Decker for his advice. He told me to send Dr. Schulman a letter making it clear that if I had no response within fifteen days, I would conclude that he "approved my study and permitted me to submit it for publication." And that's exactly what I did. When the deadline was up, I sent off my study for approval and publication. It was accepted by *The American Journal of Medicine* with high commendation. When it was published, I thought it would be only right to go and see Dr. Schulman and give him a reprint. He received me cordially and congratulated me on the strength of my character.

In the fall of 1977, Giorgos Chrousos called me. He was looking for a fellowship in clinical immunology. He wanted to work at the NIH. I knew Giorgos from when he was a student. He too was a sub-assistant many years after I was in Professor Papavassileiou's microbiology lab. A cum laude medical school graduate, extensively schooled in Ancient Greek letters, he was extremely introverted and courteous. He had written his first two scientific articles with me. In June 1978, he was finishing two years of training in pediatrics at Bellevue Hospital, which belongs to the New York University Medical School. I arranged for Giorgos to meet with the directors of various immunology laboratories. He finally found a post at the National Institute of Child Health and Human Development. He was hired as a fellow in endocrinology. After his specialization in endocrinology, he remained at the NIH for many years. He moved up through all the academic ranks. He was director of the pediatric endocrinology branch. He became an internationally recognized and highly accomplished clinical researcher. In the early 2000s, he was elected professor and chairman of the Department of Pediatrics at the Athens University Medical School.

In January 1978, our family was graced with a new member. An heir was born named Thucydides: a roly-poly, lively, and talkative baby. He spoke very quickly. Everyone said he took after me. Thucydides went back to Greece at the age of five. He was too young to start school in America. In Greece, he was a very good student, spoke flawless English and French, was a first-rate athlete, and received many awards in mathematics. He took part in many competitions run by the Hellenic Mathematical Society. He performed outstandingly. He got all the way to the Olympiad. He decided to become an engineer. I had secretly hoped he would become a doctor. I believed that suited him, because he possessed great sensitivity, was interested in helping the weak, and was very intelligent and deeply inquisitive. After completing his graduate studies in the UK, he decided to return to Ioannina, our home city. "I want to offer something to our place of origin and at the same time have a good quality life. In Ioannina everything is close: the mountains for extreme sports, the rivers for rafting, and in summer the Ionian Sea," he told me. Since that time, he has been living and working in Ioannina. He has also taken a great interest in improving the standard of living of his compatriots, and particularly in protecting the environment. I think that this may soon lead to his becoming involved in local politics, perhaps more successfully so than his father.

The publications of our studies were fast increasing in quality and number. My reputation as a clinical researcher was constantly growing. I took part in annual conferences of rheumatology, immunology, and internal medicine by presenting original research work. I was an invited speaker at various schools across the country. I was sought after by many medical schools in America. They would invite me for an interview to evaluate me, or for me to evaluate them so that they might hire me as a professor. It is a rule of thumb in the U.S., in order to hire a professor, to thoroughly study his qualifications and his personality. Unfortunately, in our country, this mentality, which leads to the choice of the most qualified candidate, usually for a university position, does not exist. In medical schools in Greece, the professorial positions are taken by individuals who have been serving the medical school for many years, or relatives and friends of the professors. The research and teaching abilities of the candidates are hardly taken into consideration. Nepotism is the order of the day.

During my visits to varied medical schools in America, I normally gave two talks, one on my clinical studies and another on my research. I would meet with the entire teaching and research staff of each department. I would visit the research laboratories and inspect the equipment, the staff, and their capabilities. None of the departments I visited, however, was as academically sound as those at the NIH. For me to change jobs, meant that something really exciting had to come up. Among the hospitals that I visited were the Hospital for Special Surgery, Cornell University Medical School, in New York, NY, the Good Samaritan Hospital, Johns Hopkins University Medical School, in Baltimore, Maryland, the Medical Center of the University of Colorado Medical School, in Denver, Colorado, and others.

Of the visits I made, one has stayed quite vivid in my mind: my visit to the medical school of Virginia University in Charlottesville, Virginia. The chairman of the internal medicine department was Professor John Davis III. His research centered on the pathogenesis of rheumatoid arthritis. He was looking for a professor with clinical and research interests in autoimmune rheumatic diseases. I had been recommended as a possible candidate, and it was suggested that he invite me for an interview. He was waiting for me at the train station. I arrived in the afternoon. He greeted me and invited me to dinner at his house, where he lived with his wife. When we arrived at the house, Mrs. Davis did the interview. She asked me for details about my family: my wife's profession, my children's ages, our extracurricular interests, and many other things. The professor retired to the kitchen. He was preparing dinner: salad, steaks, dessert, and, after the meal, coffee.

The next morning, before we went to the medical school, Professor Davis took me on a tour of the city and showed me its monuments, theater, and museums. The last stop was the cemetery. He wanted to show me the graves of his ancestors: John Davis I, physician and university professor; John Davis II, physician and university professor. After the talks, the interviews, and a visit to the department and its research labs, I made the trip back home. I was not enthusiastic about what I had seen: limited research space, not much equipment, and colleagues with no special interest in research. On the train, I had already made up my mind. This medical school was not for me.

4.3 Meeting Another Giant of Medicine

In the spring of 1978, while I was attending the Arthritis Branch patients' ward, I had the unique opportunity to meet with a giant of medicine, Professor Jan Gösta Waldenström. This prominent physician-scientist had described the hematologic disorders

Macroglobulinemia and hyperglobulinemic purpura, two pathologic entities which still bear his name.

The news that the renowned physician will visit us spread around the NIH campus like the wind. His visit to the clinical center of the NIH, for one month, was financed by the International Fogarty Center. His program included personal meetings with many researchers, who worked in similar fields to his own scientific interests. They had the opportunity to discuss with him their research findings and their plans for further work. He was carefully listening and his suggestions were very valuable. I remember, very vividly, my first meeting with Waldenström in my small office, adjacent to my laboratory. I remember him as if it was yesterday. At first sight, his noble, built posture, his appealing look, and his professional European style combined with his reputation made me feel like a schoolboy meeting a famous teacher. I presented our findings of two ongoing projects studied at that time: the presence of circulating Interferon in the blood of active systemic autoimmune patients and the occurrence of activated polyclonal and monoclonal B-lymphocytes in the blood and bone marrow of patients with Sjögren's syndrome. Professor Waldenström's interest focused on the activation of B-lymphocytes in systemic autoimmune disease. His comments and suggestions during the presentation of our study results and his very pertinent questions revealed a physician with well-rounded knowledge, not only in clinical medicine, but also in the pathogenetic mechanisms which are responsible for the development of autoimmune diseases. He put forth an argument on the ongoing theory at that time, according to which, chronicity of B-lymphocyte activation, in a genetically predisposed individual, was leading to malignant B-lymphocyte transformation. As a matter of fact, he raised some very interesting questions: "Does the chronic B-lymphocyte activation constitute the leading cause of that transformation in patients with Sjögren's syndrome?", and if this is the case: "Why then only a low percentage of these patients develop lymphoid malignancy and not the majority of them?". It took decades of research in our laboratory to find an answer to his question. In fact, our studies confirmed that Sjögren's syndrome patients who will develop lymphoid malignancy have clinical, laboratory, immunological, and molecular characteristics from the day of the disease's diagnosis.

Moreover, Professor Waldenström participated in outpatient and inpatient rounds and all of us, from senior to junior researchers, were excited to see him in action. Being responsible for the inpatient autoimmune rheumatic disease patients treated on the ninth floor of the NIH clinical center, I had the opportunity to round with Professor Waldenström. Our director, another great clinician, John L. Decker Jr, indicated the patients we should present to Waldenström. The whole team (two physicians in training and I) prepared a very detailed presentation of these cases. We were ready to respond to any possible questions our distinguished visitor might ask us. The cases were presented one after the other. Our visitor asked questions, spotted quickly the patients' problems, and made all the necessary recommendations. It was clear from his face's expression that the answers he got to his comments or questions satisfied him.

What did we gain from the inpatient and outpatient case presentations to Professor Waldenström?: (a) his empathetic approach to patients, (b) how up-to-date an academic physician should be, even in his retirement years, (c) the diagnostic and prognostic value of immunologic tests and their value for the patients' response to therapy, and last but not the least, (d) the necessity of applying patients' therapy on the basis of double-blinded controlled therapeutic trials whenever this is feasible.

At the end of his visit, he delivered a lecture in the central "Masur" auditorium of the NIH clinical center, during which he summarized his whole life research accomplishments. The amphitheater was packed and the questions, raised by the audience, were coming out thick and fast. We all wanted to take advantage of Waldenström's experience and wisdom.

This story depicts how a famous medical institute, by organizing exceptional meetings with the "Giants" of Medicine and Biology, can offer great opportunities to its junior and senior staff members to broaden their scientific knowledge.

4.4   Advisor and Coordinator of Greek Colleagues

In early July 1978, Giorgos Chrousos moved to Washington with his wife, Julie, a classmate of his and, like him, a very good student. In her first two years in New York, she worked first as a volunteer and then as an intern in the Department of Pediatrics at Bellevue Hospital. When I met her, I was impressed by her serious personality and her keen desire to continue her medical education. She wanted to become an ophthalmologist. I arranged an interview for her with the Director of the National Institute of Eye Diseases, Robert Nusssenblatt. I worked very closely with him, because he studied autoimmune diseases of the eyes. His meeting with Julie convinced him that she was qualified to work with him, and he offered her a position. Her entire disposition changed. She became a happy person, with a strong desire to soak up new knowledge. Her conscientious and successful tenure at the Institute of Eye Diseases gave her the qualifications she needed. She was soon accepted for specialization in ophthalmology. She was considered one of the finest and most well-informed residents in the educational system of the hospitals of Georgetown University Medical School. Julie quickly rose through the ranks at that university. She became a professor of ophthalmology. She is a specialist in pediatric ophthalmology and neuro-ophthalmology. Whenever I visited Georgetown University Hospital, I was delighted to see the corridor walls adorned with the awards she earned every year as a first-rate university teacher. Today, she is the director of a modern ophthalmological center in Athens, with staff that cover the entire gamut of ophthalmological diseases. Julie and Giorgos were like members of our household during all the years we lived in America. Thucydides was always thrilled when "Gogos" came to visit.

In the fall of 1978, there was a knock on the door of my laboratory and a young Greek colleague appeared. His name was Nikos Pavlidis. He was jaunty, curly-haired, and dark-skinned. In spite of the short time he had been in America, he was dressed like a Greek-American. After we had known each other for some time, I learned that his clothes were from Brazil. His mother-in-law's sister, Auntie, as he called her, had a clothing factory there. Nikos' clothes were not exactly a perfect fit. But Auntie's donations helped supplement the low income of this research fellow at the National Cancer Institute. Nikos wanted to work with me as a clinical fellow. He was already a research fellow at the experimental carcinogenesis laboratory at the National Cancer Institute, which was directed by Michael Syrigos, a Greek-American. In that lab, Nikos was studying the role of macrophages in carcinogenesis. He was an enthusiastic researcher on macrophages. He had published a good number of studies, but he had grown tired of experiments on guinea pigs. He wanted to be exposed to the beauty of internal medicine and clinical research. His maturity, self-confidence, and the coherence with which he presented his scientific thinking and aspirations convinced me that I should hire him.

I talked his candidacy over with Dr. Decker. He gave me the green light. Nikos was hired in our section. He became my shadow. He followed my every medical activity in the outpatient clinic for autoimmune rheumatic disease. He also participated in the diagnosis and therapy of hospitalized patients on the ninth-floor ward. To help him gain additional experience in medicine, I would also take him with me, as a volunteer, when I was working at night in the emergency room in Southeast Community Hospital, Washington D.C. His amiable, kind, and refined personality helped him make friends with many of the fellows in our branch (Photo 4.10). His masculine good looks attracted every type of woman. He was the "Clark Gable" of our section.

Three other young Greeks had come to America with Nikos, also with a desire to advance themselves, to refine their medical and molecular knowledge, and to add to it. They were Siphys Papamatthiakis, Vasilis Papadimitriou, and Eleni Savaki. Syphis was studying macrophages with Nikos. Vasilis was working on understanding the mechanisms that permitted a foreign implant, like an embryo, to stay in a mother's womb without being rejected. He hoped that if he could understand those mechanisms, he could use them to forestall the rejection of foreign transplanted implants. His passion, however, was to uncover the molecular mechanisms that cause arterial hypertension. He shared his aspirations with me. I introduced him to the eminent researcher on hypertension, Dr. Jim Fries, who was working at the Veterans Administration Hospital. Fries hired him, and there Vasilis began his successful academic

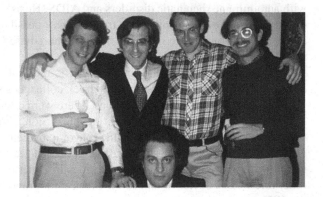

Photo 4.10 With clinical associates (from left to right): David Finbloom, author, Huib Dinant, Daniel Magilavy and Nikos Pavlidis (front)

career. Eleni was training in neurophysiology under the famous researcher Maxine Singer.

I became good friends with those young colleagues. I was their advisor in internal medicine and research. They were my teachers in Marxist ideology and the European Communist movement. They are all successful educators and researchers today. Eleni and Syphis are professors at the University of Crete, and Nikos at the University of Ioannina Medical School, while Vasilis is a professor at the Georgetown University Medical School in Washington, D.C.

At the NIH, three more Greeks held high-ranking clinical and research positions: the neuroimmunologist Marinos Dalakas, the neuroradiologist Nikos Patronas, and the clinical biochemist Nikos Papadopoulos. Marinos, an excellent clinician, was a well-known researcher of autoimmune, neuromuscular illness. He was an introvert and a loner who kept apart from the Greeks. We kept up a friendly and professional relationship, and we had many common research interests. He was elected professor of neurology at the Athens University Medical School but his active presence in the medical school was periodic and not very effective.

Nikos Patronas was a congenial, kindhearted person. He did whatever he could to help his fellow Greeks. He was the best of all the Greeks I met in America. He continued his successful academic career at the NIH.

Nikos Papadopoulos, who was some years older than the rest of us, had been of great help to me, along with his colleague Yiannis Kintzios, in the early days when I was settling in America. He had come back from Greece and was the director of the chemistry laboratory, part of the clinical pathology laboratories at the NIH Clinical Center. He was like a second father to me. His wife, Aliki, and his children treated me like a close friend or a relative. Nikos was always pleased with my progress and closely followed the developments in my career as a clinician and researcher. Whenever I presented my clinical or research data, he was always the first to arrive, and would sit in the front row of the lecture hall. His scientific interest was focused on the role of lipoproteins in atherosclerosis. He had developed a sensitive elec-trophoretic method, and he was the first person to describe type III hyperlipidemia. In addition, his sensitive electrophoretic technique enabled us to study, in the blood and in cerebrospinal fluids, the products of premalignant B-lymphocytes of patients with autoimmune rheumatic disorders and AIDS. He assumed the role of champion of the younger Greek scientists. He tried in every possible way to support scientists newly arrived from Greece. He was the one who advised me to hire Nikos Pavlidis as a fellow.

My own contribution to the Greek scientific medical community was as a coor-dinator. My office was always open to Greek colleagues seeking advice or help for personal, family, or professional reasons. There were often quarrels in our close-knit community. They were all intelligent people. I don't know what pushed them to want to outdo one another. I played the role of a mediator in their trivial, ego-fueled clashes. I believed that we should all be united. If we wanted to succeed, we had to follow in the footsteps of other minorities in America and learn from them. My other role was as doctor of uninsured Greek immigrants, whom I treated for free at the NIH.

4.5 An Opportunity to Repatriate

In the winter of 1978, some excellent news arrived. Two new medical schools in Greece, belonging to the Universities of Ioannina and Patras, announced openings for the position of professor and chairman of internal medicine. I considered myself advanced enough to apply for this position. I believed that my days as an immigrant had served their purpose, that is, to help me develop as a physician, teacher, and researcher. The idea that I could return to the place where I was born, raised, and had my first lessons in medicine, as a professor in charge of creating a university-level department of internal medicine, filled me with joy, happiness, and hope and seemed like a dream coming true. I was sure that if they gave me that position, I would help put Ioannina on the map of medical schools that produced excellent young physicians, as well as original and groundbreaking work. I imagined that the new knowledge that would be generated by my department would be on a par with what is produced at the best-known medical centers abroad. I envisioned attracting excellently trained specialists in internal medicine and building a department together that would serve to treat patients in our area. I was convinced that the educational program we would implement would create excellently trained young physicians of high moral caliber, with great sensitivity to the problems of ailing patients. All of this was going around in my head before I even saw the electors, and without knowing anything about their intentions. But my enthusiasm was so great that nothing could discourage me and my dreams. I prepared my curriculum vitae, along with copies of my research papers and, with my father's help, I submitted my application.

I had to inform the directors at the NIH about my decision and ask them for letters of reference. The first person I visited was Dr. Decker. After hearing all my plans, he remained silent for a minute or two and looked at me. Then, with a stentorian voice and an imperious expression, he said to me: "Have you really thought this through? You're going to cut short a brilliant career, now that you've reached the height of your powers, to transfer to a medical school no one has heard of? What are they offering you to go there?" That great researcher and teacher of medicine could not get inside my mind. He couldn't understand that I had gone to America to better myself. I hadn't immigrated in order to stay forever in my new country. My own country was pulling me back like a powerful magnet. I explained to him that for me America was an excellent place to develop scientifically, but that I had never planned to spend my whole life in a foreign country. The opportunity that had come up just then was unique, because I could return to my country. "If they elect me," I told him,"it will be a chance to set up a department of internal medicine with high academic standards and a research center that will soon be producing original research." He did not seem convinced by my arguments. "Since you're so anxious to return to your country, I cannot stop you, nor do I want to. But I strongly suggest you stay here. You are making great progress, and I'm sure that very soon you will be in the seat I now occupy." I thanked him and I assured him that, if I was accepted in Greece, he would see that my department would soon be producing innovative research.

The second person I had to see and bring up-to-date was Dr. Fauci. He would not even listen to my decision. He thought I had suddenly gone out of my mind. He tried his best to make me reconsider. He offered me the position of clinical director of the National Institute of Allergic and Infectious diseases. But I had made up my mind. There was nothing that could change it. I asked him to write me a detailed letter of recommendation, analyzing my clinical, teaching, and research skills, and also mentioning the maturity and administrative ability I showed, a prerequisite for the position of professor and chairman of the Department of Internal Medicine at the University of Ioannina. "I'll do it," he told me, "but with a heavy heart. I'm afraid that this decision of yours may retard or even destroy your academic career."

The news that I was trying to return to Greece circulated around the institutes like lightning. No one agreed with my decision. But I was sticking by it.

I made a program to see all eleven electors for the Chair of internal medicine at the University of Ioannina. Fortunately, most of them were in America. Giorgos Rallis, Minister of Education and Religious Affairs at that time, had made a special legal framework for the new medical schools. He didn't want them to be extensions of the old medical schools, but to be hubs for attracting new brainpower from the Greek Diaspora. The electoral bodies were composed of experts in the field, half of whom were Greek professors in foreign universities. The electors for the Chair of internal medicine at the medical school of the University of Ioannina were the following professors of internal medicine in America: Giorgos Bousvaros (New York), Athanasios Theologidis (Minneapolis), and Georgios Emmanouilidis (Los Angeles); and from Greece, Georgios Daïkos (Athens), Georgios Merikas (Athens), and Georgios Tsourouktsoglou (Thessaloniki). The electoral body was completed by the four newly elected chairmen of basic science: Othonas Kotoulas (anatomy), Orestis Tsolas (biochemistry), Gerasimos Pagoulatos (biology), and Giorgos Kallistratos (physiology). All were Greeks who had studied for many years abroad and made significant scientific contributions to their fields. The chairman of the electoral body was Professor Vasilios Staikos, from the Department of Mathematics of the University of Ioannina.

There were eleven candidates for the Chair of internal medicine at the medical school of the University of Ioannina: nine docents from the Universities of Athens and Thessaloniki, and two Diaspora Greeks, Dr. Giorgos Tolis and I. The interviews with the professors of internal medicine from America were a feast of exchanging information. They studied my academic progress with great interest, asked about my plans for the future, tried to flesh out my ideas for the development of the new Department of Internal Medicine, were interested in my thinking, and generously offered their experienced opinions about my possible return to Greece. In stark contrast, the interviews with the majority of the professors of internal medicine in Greece were formal and polite, without any serious analysis of my qualifications as a candidate. It appears that the job of elector was a chore rather than a pleasure. They did not appear to fully understand the responsibilities entailed by the function of an elector.

My interview with Professor Tsourouktsoglou was a tragic comedy. The appointment was at 7:30 a.m. I took the Olympic Airways morning flight to Thessaloniki and at 7:15 I was outside his office. At 7:30 he arrived. He greeted me and told me to wait in his office, because he had to attend to a serious matter. He put on his white doctor's gown and left. He was taking a long time to return, and I was bored. I had spent the time looking at the archaic books in his dusty bookcase. I decided it was time to see where the professor was. I stepped out of the office and a surprise was waiting for me in the corridor of the clinic. The professor was chasing the visitors out of the patients' ward. I asked him politely to please give me a bit of time for our interview. I had to catch a plane back to Athens so as not to miss my flight to America. We went into his office, and there another surprise awaited me. He asked me if I was a clinician because, as he told me, he didn't understand any of my papers. I answered him at once: "Please ask one of your residents to present a patient's case, so you can evaluate and see for yourself my differential diagnostic and my diagnostic skills and my abilities as a clinician." "It is not our practice to do that," he said. I left Thessaloniki in very low spirits, feeling certain that that particular elector was not going to support me.

This was offset by my meeting with Professor Daïkos, which improved my disposition considerably. He was logical, sharp-minded, and courteous, and he wanted to study the qualifications of the candidates before making a final decision. Among the basic scientists I visited were Orestes Tsolas, in New York. The interview took place in the presence of the famous Professor B. Horecker, director of the Roche Translational and Clinical Research Center. The interview was like a small-scale scientific symposium. I presented the results of my studies. I explained my plans for future research, and I elaborated on my hopes to create a model internal medicine department. I believe they were pleased. I returned to Washington satisfied and happy. I visited the other professors from the Ioannina University Medical School, in Greece. My interview with Othon Kotoulas was formal, in spite of his many years of training abroad. His time at the Athens University Medical School had irreparably suffused him with the mentality of a conservative health official. My meeting with Gerasimos Pagoulatos filled me with anxiety and sadness. He was concerned about my reputation of not being a clinician. He believed that a professor of internal medicine at the University of Ioannina should be someone who had been working for many years in an internal medicine department. My meeting with the late Giorgos Kallistratos was pleasant. It had nothing to do with my candidacy, however. He described to me at length a program of his for planting trees on every balcony and terrace of every apartment building in the city of Ioannina, and adding various species of fish and eels to Lake Pamvotis.

The electors of the Ioannina University Medical School encouraged me to meet with a non-tenured professor of medical physics at the medical school, Dimitris Glaros. He was not a member of the electoral body, but from what they said he appeared to be the heart and soul of the medical school.

Our meeting reminded me of an interview held abroad with a candidate for a professorship. Dimitris was tall, courteous, amiable, and outspoken, which made his beliefs apparent: "The Ioannina University Medical School will become a prototype for higher education in our country." He later became a very successful rector of the university.

The electors' evaluation of the candidates for the Chair of internal medicine was finalized and submitted. I was first on the list. The election was set for March 25, 1979. Several days ahead of time I took the plane to Greece. I wanted to be in Ioannina on the day of the election. I met again with as many electors as were available. From what they said, it looked like they would elect me or Giorgos Tolis. During the election itself, the vigorous support of Professor Daïkos and the professors of internal medicine from America gave me an absolute majority: nine votes out of eleven. Professor Tsourouktsoglou voted for Giorgos Tolis, and Professor Merikas voted for one of his colleagues. Many years later, after I had given a talk at a Greek symposium, Professor Merikas came up to me, took me aside, and had the kindness to congratulate me for my teaching abilities and the scientific soundness of my talk, and he confessed to me that he had misgivings about not having voted for me for the Chair of internal medicine at the Ioannina University Medical School. He told me that he wanted to correct this mistake. Several months later, he notified me that I was unanimously elected corresponding member of the Academy of Athens.

I was now professor-elect and director of the Chair of internal medicine at the Ioannina University Medical School. My election made me happy and filled me with hope for the future. Without wasting any time, I threw myself into my work. I had to select textbooks for my students. I wanted to prepare an up-to-date post-graduate training program for interns and residents in the department I was taking over. At that time, the patient wards of the Department of Internal Medicine were located at the Hatzicostas Hospital. From the time of the election until the swearing in of the professor, at least six months are needed. So, I had plenty of time to complete my work at the NIH.

In the spring of 1979, several months before my return to Greece to assume my professorship, another young couple, both Greek colleagues, knocked at the door of my laboratory at the NIH. It was Giorgos and Maria Tsokos. Giorgos, an internist with experience in immunology, had worked in the immunology laboratory at Agios Savvas Hospital, in Athens, directed by Dr. Mihalis Papamihail. Maria was a pathologist. Both wished to continue their studies. Giorgos, a nervous sort who spoke very quickly and tended to be over-assertive, tried to convince me to hire him as a fellow. Maria was unassuming, quiet, and conservatively dressed. It seems she was the one giving the orders in the family. I explained to them that I had no open position. I did promise them, however, that I would try to find them a place in another laboratory. Giorgos asked me to give him a research project to work on until he found a position. I suggested that he study the clinical, immunological, and pathological picture of myositis, an inflammation of the muscles that appears in patients with systemic lupus erythematosus. He was a hard worker, persistent and thorough, and he soon collected the information. The study was completed, and it was accepted for publication by the *Journal of the American Medical Association*. It was not long before their problems were settled once and for all. Giorgos became a fellow with the nephrologist Jim Bellow and Maria with Jose Costa, director of the pathology laboratory of the NIH Clinical Center and an internationally recognized researcher on vasculitis.

That summer, two medical school students came to work as volunteers in my department. One was a Greek-American named Spyros Lazarou, a graduate of Johns Hopkins University Medical School. "I'm your compatriot," he said to me in broken Greek. "Nikos Papadopoulos sent me to do research with you. I would like a clinical subject to study." I assigned him to study vasculitis in patients with Sjögren's syndrome. Maria Tsokos helped him substantially in that study. By the end of the summer, the study was ready. Spyros went on to do his training in surgery and, in particular, plastic surgery. After many years of training, he was repatriated to Greece. He is now considered the most respectable and capable plastic surgeon in Athens. He has a private practice. But he has never stopped selflessly alleviating human suffering, and voluntarily performing surgery in many underdeveloped countries. He fulfilled his father's wish and desire to return to his homeland.

The other fourth-year medical school student was the Anglo-Saxon John Gallagher. Dr. Decker introduced me to him. He studied the clinical and laboratory picture of herpes zoster in patients with systemic lupus erythematosus. So, in the summer of 1979, my rather small laboratory was busy as a beehive, filled with many people, all working hard, productive, and anxious to learn new things.

Come fall, I was back at the NIH, and two more delightful things happened. Dr. Decker was worried about my decision to return to Greece. He called me to his office. He reiterated his fears, and he gave me an unexpected gift. He told me: "I want you to keep your position at the NIH. But because I can't keep you in the position you now hold, I am going to appoint you as a clinical consultant. You'll spend two or three months a year here at our branch. The position will be activated whenever you return. You will serve as the attending physician of a clinical team of physicians at the patient ward of our institute and, at the same time, with biological material that you will bring from Greece, or by reviewing the medical records of the patients at the institute, you will be able to continue your research. If you don't make it in your country, the institute will always be waiting for you with open arms." I cannot describe the emotions that came over me: relief, joy, assurance, and pride.

The second honor that was awaiting me was that they assigned me to coordinate a clinical conference at the NIH on Sjögren's syndrome. The speakers at the meeting were all the researchers we had collaborated with to better understand that syndrome: A. Fauci, S. Katz, M. Frank, T. Chused, T. Lawley, and M. Hamburger. The proceedings of the meeting were published in Annals of Internal Medicine. That publication remained the cornerstone of the work of many other researchers studying Sjögren's syndrome, for many decades.

Because of my clinical and research work on so many fronts, I didn't realize how much time had passed. In September 1979, I received the official Greek Government Gazette in the mail, listing my appointment as "professor and chair of internal medicine and director of the internal medicine department of the Hatzicostas General State Hospital in Ioannina." I had to be sworn in within two months. We took our oath back then with the minister of education. I decided to fulfill that obligation during the last ten days of October. The swearing-in ceremony was magisterial. It kept you both conscious and confident of the fact that you were about to assume an office of the highest order. After I was sworn in, I had the right, as a permanent resident abroad, to take a six-month leave of absence to complete my relocation. But I was bothered by the thought that my medical students had already reached their third year of studies and there was no professor to teach them about the mechanisms that cause diseases and the techniques for examining and communicating with patients. Through my attitude and through example, it was my duty to teach them the importance of empathy and responsibility when examining patients. So, I decided not to take advantage of the legal options for postponement at my disposal and take up my post in January 1980. I was very pleased that the time had come to offer all my expertise to my country of origin, a goal I had for so long envisioned.

During the few days I spent in Ioannina, I intended to gather information on how the department I was taking over functioned, what the scientific level was, and the future plans of the physicians working in it. But above all, I wanted to meet the students and discuss with them the demands of our profession, and familiarize them with the educational program I had organized, and inspire in them a love for our field of study.

The dean and the administrative secretary welcomed me. At the time the administrative offices of the medical school were located in an apartment building in the center of Ioannina, just opposite the courthouse. The dean soon expressed his apprehension concerning my deferred return. "The students are waiting for you," said the dean. "I have decided to return in January," I told him. His expression turned calm and relieved. "Many of them would like to meet you right now," he told me, and without giving me a chance to answer, he informed me that such a meeting could take place the same or the next day, when the students had no other educational activities. A date was set. A day was also arranged for me to visit the hospital wards, meet the staff, and see how well it was functioning.

The meeting with the students took place at the Kamperio Cultural Center in the center of Ioannina. This was the amphitheater that was used for teaching pre-clinical students. I remember that meeting quite clearly. The students were really paying attention; they hung on my every word, as the saying goes, anxious to see what the new professor had to say. I could see from the puzzled expressions on their faces what they were thinking, as though they were asking me, "When are we starting classes?".

After briefly describing my life to them, I let them know I would be starting to teach in January. Next, I tried to sum up and describe not only the beauty of medical art and science, but also the obligations and responsibilities entailed by our profession. "Medicine," I told them "requires servants with a limitless predisposition for hard work, responsibility, compassion for the ill, generosity, benevolence, selflessness, and immeasurable respect for one's patients. Above all else, however, our profession demands, due to continued new developments, that you keep informed and study hard, so that you are capable of providing the most up-to-date diagnosis and effective therapy. But aside from these inflexible prerequisites, medicine needs people who are passionate about it. That is to say, it needs lovers: people who do not feel like they are working, but are eager to go to work in the morning as though it were a hobby." I closed that short introduction by encouraging them to ask questions continually, and not to be afraid that their questions might not be smart. "There are no stupid questions," I said. "There are only people who are not smart enough to ask questions and therefore never learn."

As I was told later by one of those students who still works with me today, it was the first time that those students realized that to become a professor of medicine you did not have to be advanced in age. They were not aware that the criteria for electing a professor are not vague descriptions of one's experience, but rather clear, up-to-date, well-documented knowledge and scientific contributions.

During my visit to the hospital's medical wards, there were more surprises in store for me. I was amazed at the extensive length of hospital stays for insignificant problems, the lack of a plan to treat the patient, the undocumented therapeutic interventions, and the poor medical care. The most amazing thing, however, was that there were no medical records for the patients. Instead of a medical file, they used a sheet of paper attached to a small tin board hung at the foot of the patients' beds. On these, they recorded the patient's blood pressure, pulse, temperature, as well as the results of a few laboratory tests, whenever they were performed.

When the visit was over, I spoke personally to every member of the staff and the residents. All of them, together, told me they wanted to stay in their positions and continue working under my supervision. One of the major responsibilities of the head of a medical department was to inspire the young physicians to see the beauty of our profession, to create in them the selfless desire to give to others, along with respect for the patient, and to teach them to dream; to dream about a bright future full of knowledge that would accord them diagnostic and therapeutic competence along with the inexpressible satisfaction of exercising their profession. I wanted to teach them to pursue excellence, to pursue the impossible, and to pursue all their goals. I also had to teach them and convince them of the necessity to create and keep medical records for every patient. I suggested to them that we translate the medical records of the Georgetown University Medical center. "We'll have it ready when you return in January," they told me all together.

I went back to America for about two months. I had to resign from the section. During those two months, I prepared the courses in pathophysiology and the practical exercises to teach medical students how to take the patient's history and perform a complete physical examination.

Chapter 5
Chair of Internal Medicine, Ioannina University Medical School

5.1 Assuming the Chair

In January of 1980, I assumed my duties as professor of the Chair of internal medicine and chairman of one of the two departments of Internal Medicine at the Hatzicostas State Hospital, a hospital with no academic tradition or technical and material infrastructure, and which was inadequate even for a regional hospital. It was the former sanatorium of Ioannina. Several of the departments of the regional hospital were redesignated as university departments.

Aside from the position of professor, the department of Internal Medicine had seven more positions: one consultant, two lecturers, two university-level staff members, and two secretaries. All were vacant, ready to be announced. The former government-run department of Internal Medicine was staffed by the director already working there, two attending physicians, five residents, the head nurse, and ten more nurses. All employees, who were already serving at the government internal medicine department, remained in their posts as staff members of the university internal medicine department.

The patients were crammed into three wards meant to hold eight patients each, but actually housing ten or twelve. There were also two wards for six patients each that mostly held eight or ten patients, two single rooms, the director's office, the hospital staff office, the nurses' station, and a small room where the night-shift doctors slept. None of the hospital wards had a bathroom. There were common bathrooms for all the patients in one place on the floor where the wards of the department were.

An important section of the department was the hemodialysis unit. It was operated by the nurses and a physician of the internal medicine department, who had had a few months of training in a hemodialysis unit of the Athens State Hospital. I assigned the former director of the department of Internal Medicine to be in charge of the hemodialysis unit. The state cardiology section and the coronary care unit voluntarily became sections of the university internal medicine department. In this way, both the medical students and the residents had a chance to also be trained in acute and chronic heart problems. So I began, little by little, to refashion the Chair of internal

© The Author(s), under exclusive license to Springer Nature Switzerland AG 2022
H. M. Moutsopoulos, *Passion for Excellence*, Springer Biographies,
https://doi.org/10.1007/978-3-031-14128-7_5

medicine into a functional department of Internal Medicine, the goal of which was excellent care for patients and satisfactory training for medical students and residents during their specialization program.

One of my main concerns was to inspire the young physicians, interns, and residents whom I took into the department as trainees to appreciate the beauty of our profession, to create in them the need to improve their medical knowledge by studying the literature on the basis of their patients' problems, to offer empathetic care to their patients, and to keep the patients' medical records updated. I spoke to each of them personally.

The students in the medical school were now in their third year. Fortunately, there were not too many of them, only about a hundred, most of whom were very eager to learn. Until January there would be no professor of internal medicine. So, during the remainder of the academic year we would have to cover a whole year's material in pathophysiology, plus teach them how to take patients' medical histories and perform a thorough physical examination.

I began classes immediately. At that time, I taught in an auditorium at the Kamperio Cultural Center. It was a building with roomy, sun-filled halls in the center of Ioannina, three kilometers away from the hospital. Lectures were held in the morning, while clinical tutorials on patient care for students, in teams of five or six, took place in the afternoon. During the hours in between, on many afternoons until late at night, I had plenty of time to supervise the care of my patients, to organize the functioning of my department, and to participate in the administration of the medical school and keep myself up-to-date on the latest medical developments by studying the best-known journals in our field.

One of the two government-appointed attending physicians soon submitted his resignation. He couldn't keep up with the demanding rhythms of a university internal medicine department. But he found the environment in the Department of Experimental Physiology both accommodating and comfortable, and he soon joined the ranks of its faculty members. After only two or three months of training abroad, he was promoted to professor of experimental physiology. Unfortunately, this is the sad reality in many laboratories and departments of the medical schools in our country.

The vacant position of the government-appointed attending physician was announced and filled in short order. We had substantial and consistent help in our efforts from the Minister of Health, Spyros Doxiades. The new attending physician, Dr. Petros Avgerinos, had received excellent training in internal medicine in the United Kingdom. Completely loyal, good-natured, hard-working, unusually courteous, and extremely eager to augment his knowledge, he soon fell in line with the demands of a university internal medicine department. For the position of consultant, I had selected an internist-hematologist, Dr. Garoufallia Kokkini. She was a fellow in hematology at the Rockefeller University Medical School, in America. She was a hard worker, dedicated to her field, excellently trained in internal medicine and in hematology, demanding of herself and of others, completely selfless, and an unusually good teacher with an unparalleled predisposition to generate new biomedical knowledge. After an extensive interview, we decided that she would be a valuable member of the newly established university internal medicine department. She was given the position of consultant, a university position that on the one hand was clearly higher than that of a lecturer, and on the other hand would give her the right to be the director of the hospital blood bank at the same time. A hematologist without a laboratory is like an internist without a stethoscope. She soon organized a contemporary hematology lab, while at the same time she took over the duties of attending physician and teacher of our medical students.

Having such close contact with the students quickly made me able to pick out those students with a strong interest in medicine. One of the honor students, Dimitris Boumpas, took on the job of helping me translate the *Bates' Guide to Physical Examination and History Taking,* a clear, concise, simple and brief handbook, with pictures, drawings, and charts. With the intensive and diligent efforts of the Litsas Publishing Co., the handbook was ready for the 1981–82 academic year. It became a bestseller at the time. The Patras University Medical School also adopted it as a textbook. Dimitris, after many years of training in America, returned to become a professor at the Athens University Medical School.

Another goal of mine was to teach the residents to perform invasive procedures, such as inserting a catheter in a subclavian vein, doing biopsies of the liver, the peritoneum, the pleura, and the bone marrow. I had brought with me from the NIH the corresponding biopsy needles. All those procedures are still carried out successfully and with few complications, even in hospital corridors with patients on cots.

It was an absolute necessity for all interns and residents to be able to perform general urine tests and a Gram stain on the sputum and other fluids from patients with a possible infection, to determine as soon as possible the microbes responsible for the infection.

Two resident physicians quickly stood out in my mind. They had a high level of medical knowledge, they cared about their patients, they studied the patients' medical problems thoroughly, they kept up-to-date on the medical literature, and they happily and uncomplainingly passed on whatever they knew to their students. They were Nikos Akritidis and Yiannis Goudevenos. From the beginning, they acted as unpaid young faculty members to help run our department. Nikos, after successfully advancing his career, was soon appointed director of the department of Internal Medicine at the Hatzicostas Hospital. Yiannis, after four years of education in cardiology in the U.K., joined the faculty of the cardiology section of our department and soon progressed to the level of professor of cardiology.

A university internal medicine department has a three-fold purpose: high-quality patient care, teaching medical students and residents doing their specialization, and the generation of new medical knowledge. But to be productive, a university internal medicine department must have first-rate medical and nursing staff. The support and contribution of the small number of nurses under the exemplary guidance of the head nurse, Matina Agorastou, was of substantial help in raising the level of patient care. The nurses were tireless, always smiling, and eager to help their patients. The long hours and the pressures of work never got them down. They only wanted to offer their services. I had the good luck to have several nurses among those in my department who had been trained abroad. The most shining example of what a nurse should be remains that of Tereza Papadopoulou. She was working in a hospital in

Germany where she met her partner, a worker from Ioannina, and returned with him to Ioannina. She came from Croatia. She was the perfect model of a health worker completely devoted to her job. She organized the outpatient clinic for autoimmune rheumatic diseases.

The example of the nursing staff, however, seems to have annoyed others at the hospital, for whom working hours meant time to gossip and relax. Their reaction soon became apparent. Backed by sources I would rather not name, an article appeared in the local press. In it, there was an ironic reference to me stating that I had put wheels under the nurses' feet so they would be more productive. Fortunately, the local community paid no attention to such spiteful articles.

Also essential for an internal medicine department to function are fully organized and well-run diagnostic laboratories, specialized intensive care units, and sections of other branches of medicine that are run with a view toward excellence. The contribution of the university radiology laboratory under the directorship of Professor Pavlos Katsiotis played a decisive role in making our department operational. He quickly organized an exemplary radiology department. Soon afterward, he also developed an invasive radiology section and an ultrasound section, under the supervision of an unusually well-trained colleague from the U.K., Kostas Tsampoulas.

The contribution of the pathology laboratory, directed by Kostas Papadimitriou, was catalytic in improving our department's diagnostic capabilities. As he himself liked to say, the University of Ioannina department of Internal Medicine was now first-rate in invasive medical procedures. I had taught the new physicians to perform organ biopsies. The pathology laboratory was flooded with tissue samples: skin, liver, bone marrow, pleura, peritoneum, and later kidney.

In contrast, the help provided to us by the university microbiology laboratory was minimal. Unfortunately, the professor in charge, despite his long tenure abroad, had never worked in a diagnostic laboratory in a tertiary hospital. As a result, he seemed unaware that, in order to provide excellent care to patients, certain examinations had to be carried out on an emergency basis. His only interest was in not tiring his staff. We tried to make up for the deficiencies of that laboratory by creating a small-scale laboratory in one of the bathrooms on the floor where the wards of our department were located. The hospital soon procured a machine to measure arterial blood gases, and our resident physicians were trained in carrying out emergency examinations of blood smears and urine samples. We also purchased a small analyzer, which was able to measure patients' blood sugar, creatinine, and electrolytes. Necessity is the mother of invention. Garyfallia Kokkini gave us invaluable help in diagnosing diseases of the blood. She was a first-rate diagnostician of bone marrow diseases.

To boost the level of medical knowledge of the physicians in our department, we organized graduate courses from the very first months that we began functioning. Every Monday afternoon, we held a bibliographical briefing where a resident, together with an attending physician who was his supervisor, would present, analyze and discuss new developments in our field, based on information in the most prestigious journals, such as *Annals of Internal Medicine*, *The Lancet*, and *The New England Journal of Medicine*. In this way, we believed that the physicians in our department would be kept up-to-date on the latest developments. Every Wednesday, we would have a lecture by a visiting professor from another university in Greece, or from abroad. These lecturers were selected based solely on academic criteria. We did not use the podium, or the visiting lecturers as a means of promoting ourselves socially, or engaging in university politics. Every Thursday, to improve the residents' and students' abilities in differential diagnosis, we would have a clinical pathology conference, using an interesting medical case. Each case was chosen from *The New England Journal of Medicine,* and the discussion was led by an internist from our department who would use the selected case as a means of teaching pathogenesis, differential diagnosis, and treatment. Every day from 3–4 p.m., in collaboration with the university radiology laboratory, we would discuss various interesting X-rays. Due to a lack of available teaching space, these lessons were held in the chairman's office. It was tightly packed with residents from our department, physicians from other departments of the hospital, as well as nurses eager to participate in this educational endeavor. Twice a week the chairman's office also served as an outpatient clinic for autoimmune rheumatic diseases.

I made it clear to everyone from the outset that the chairman would be the model of an energetic physician. He would be the first one to arrive in the morning and the last to leave in the evening. He would always be nearby and available to them to help solve their problems, but he would demand that his assignments be carried out.

5.2   Selecting Secretaries

When you are working in the place where you were born and grew up, this is very nice on the one hand. Everywhere you go, you remember something. Everyone is a relative, a friend, or an acquaintance. Everyone thinks of you as one of theirs. Many are proud because one of their own reached the highest academic ranks. Others feel assured that their friend will take care of them if they ever need to be hospitalized. On the other hand, however, the position of professor and department chairman carries certain powers with it. Many expect their friend to help a child or grandchild, or nephew of theirs, because this type of social bargaining is rampant in our country. To be honest, I was afraid that I might be influenced in my choices of the administrative or scientific staff I was hiring, so from the very first days that I took up the post of chairman, I avoided dinners and receptions to which I was invited. The only people I went out with, on an occasional evening at some out-of-the-way restaurant, were colleagues or people I worked closely with. I was too busy with my teaching, clinical, and administrative obligations. Most of my friends and relatives forgave me for this, but others wondered if the time I spent abroad had turned me into a loner and a misanthrope. Whenever I talked to friends and relatives from Ioannina, I never failed to mention and convey the message that the only way forward for our medical school was to select for each and every position, from nurse to professor, only the best-qualified candidates. There was no other way, I proclaimed right and left, for our medical school to provide the best possible care for patients, and the best possible education for our budding young doctors, and to claim a prominent place in the international domain of medical science.

In the early months of 1980, based on the theory that whatever was from America was exceptional, I hired on a temporary work contract a Greek-American woman who had studied to be an administrative assistant. She was perfect when it came to communicating with countries abroad, but she had significant problems in her knowledge of Greek and in typing Greek documents.

Fortunately, the time went by quickly and the two positions for secretary of the Chair were announced. We had more than twenty candidates. I had the presence of mind beforehand, with two other colleagues on the board of directors of our school, to list in the announcement the qualifications for secretary: (a) high grades in high school or in secretarial school; (b) ability to type perfectly in Greek and in English; (c) ability to keep records; and (d) fluency in another language. All candidates meeting these criteria would be examined by a three-member committee to determine their proficiency in a foreign language and their ability to type a text in Greek and in English. Finally, I would interview the top four candidates and choose the best two.

I must confess that no one from Ioannina came to me about supporting specific candidates. Based on the qualifications listed in the announcement, half of the candidates were disqualified after being examined. The positions were finally given to Eleni Papa and Evangelia Papanikolaou (Photo 5.1). The criteria we used to select them proved to be accurate. We picked the two truly devoted employees who were the most anxious and willing to offer their services, with irreproachable ethics and indefatigable work habits. The departmental director and the secretaries functioned as a harmonious unit. They were only interested in promoting the progress of the internal medicine department and serving the students and the patients' needs.

Though both secretaries were of left-wing persuasions, which were typical of the political ideologies of that period, they were never caught up in party-line bickering or syndicalist activism and never got distracted from their professional obligations. Their will to work was so strong that they were more than capable of withstanding the ironic and malicious comments of the unionists in their workplace. Much time has passed since the beginning of the decade of the 1980s but, believe me, I still have

Photo 5.1 Department secretaries, Evangelia Papanikolaou and Helen Pappa

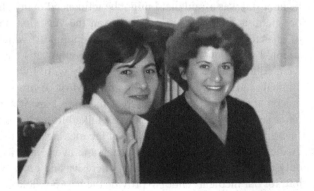

these two ladies in my mind and my heart. I care about them as much as I do about my closest friends or relatives. I am sure that they feel the same way about me.

Together, we had to take care of the pressing administrative needs of our school (hiring of administrative personnel, purchase of equipment, selection and approval of textbooks, etc.) and to arrange for the announcement of the candidacies for additional faculty members, attending physicians, interns, and residents.

5.3 And the Problems Begin

5.3.1 Side-Stepping the Law

When I was still a candidate for a professorship at the Ioannina University Medical School, I was frequently updated on the course of my candidacy by the secretary in charge of the administration of the medical school. The administration operated the same way as in medical schools in more developed countries. I was impressed by how well it was run.

During my visits to Ioannina in order to meet the electors—four professors from the medical school and the chairman of the electoral committee, Professor Vasilios Staikos from the Department of Mathematics—I became aware of how few administrative employees there were in the medical school. The administration consisted of the secretary, and two assistants, both high school graduates. My acquaintance with the secretary went back to our school days. She was a graduate of Athens University Law School. She had made it the purpose of her professional life to run the administration of the Ioannina medical school faultlessly. An active, clever woman with a strong personality, she worked endless hours to achieve her goal. I must confess that I believed my acquaintance with her was the reason for my detailed updates from the administration. I found out, however, that the other candidates were also updated regularly on the course of their candidacies. So, in fact I did not enjoy special treatment. Quite simply, the administration functioned perfectly.

The year I took up the Chair, a professor of anatomy held the position of dean. The dean's term of office was one year. He was senior to all of us. At a certain point, he had temporarily lost his Chair due to a legal appeal lodged by a fellow candidate with the Council of State. This resulted in the first deanship of the newly established medical school being held by the second in seniority professor of physiology. There was an underlying rivalry between those two senior professors. The professor of anatomy never got over the fact that he was not able to serve as the first dean of the Ioannina University Medical School.

But let's go back and look at things one by one. The Ioannina University Medical School began functioning in the academic year 1977–1978, without student laboratories, without a university hospital, and without administrative personnel. The teachers of the first-year medical students were professors of chemistry, physics, biology, and statistics from other schools of the university. The newly founded medical school had, however, accepted a rather large number of students, most of whom were extremely eager to learn. The administration of the medical school had a huge workload and was under great pressure. It had to resolve student issues, hire teaching staff, and supervise the procedures for electing permanent faculty members. All of this work was carried out by the three employees of the administration. The secretary's two assistants were working under six-month contracts. The law at that time did not permit them to be re-hired when their contracts expired. New employees had to be hired as assistants to the secretary. These new assistants had to be trained before they could perform any work. But the problems were non-stop and could not wait. The dean, in order to avoid disruption of the smooth functioning of the administration, solved this problem in an original way. He hired as new assistants of the secretary, on paper only, relatives of the old assistants, while in fact these old assistants continued working for the secretary. The professor of physiology had studied and made a career abroad. He was not familiar with the rules and regulations that governed the functioning of university medical schools in Greece. He tried, as dean, to run the school as best he could, with the best intentions and with common sense.

The following academic year, the professor of anatomy was restored to his Chair and assumed the position of dean. Thorough by nature and a proponent of the letter of the law, he discovered the violation. Instead of overlooking it, seeing as the actions of the previous dean were motivated solely by expediency and did not bring him any personal gain, but simply helped the medical school to continue running smoothly, the new dean brought the problem up at the weekly faculty meeting. It was clear that he wanted the professor of physiology to be punished. But he did not propose this, and instead tried indirectly to place the blame on the secretary of the administration of the medical school, an action that brings to mind the popular saying: "When the donkey is at fault, blame it on the saddle."

The discussions of this problem at faculty meetings made our lives miserable for many weeks. We wasted many hours discussing matters which, in America at least, had no legal basis. I tried to find the minutes of those meetings. I would have liked to reproduce those discussions here word for word, but I was unable to find them. All I found were summaries of the discussions that were not particularly enlightening. I remember that it was not until after many meetings that I began to understand the problem. I suggested to my colleagues that instead of us going on and on about it, it should be examined by a three-member committee that would perform an administrative investigation under oath. Their investigation would reveal if there was a guilty party and that party's identity. My colleagues did not agree with my proposal. It was clear that they did not want the previous dean to be held responsible. They preferred to place the blame on the secretary of the administration. They pointed out that the secretary, as a lawyer herself, should have protected the dean from this illegal administrative action. Many weeks went by, with discussion after discussion, and no significant outcome. In the end, the dean's term finished and the whole matter was forgotten, fortunately.

It is time now to confess a personal "misconduct".

Cardiac diseases are one of the commonest disorders in humans. Thus, the presence of a contemporary cardiologist in our department was of paramount importance for patient's care and the education of medical students and residents. I tried to attract a well-trained Greek cardiologist from the Diaspora who was planning to repatriate. The geographical isolation of Ioannina, however, was a serious obstacle. I couldn't find the right person.

I had two choices, either to hire someone with insufficient qualifications, or to ignore the letter of the law, of course not for my own benefit. In my own professional value system, the second choice was preferable to the first. So, what did I do? I arranged for Dr. Yiannis Goudevenos, a well-trained internist and junior staff member of the department, to be specialized in cardiology at the University Medical Center of Newcastle-upon Tyne, in the U.K.

However, he had not served in the department the necessary time required by the law in order to take a sabbatical leave of absence. Our efforts to get him a scholarship failed. As the Chairman of the department, I decided to take the responsibility and allow Yiannis, while in Newcastle, to continue drawing his salary as a university-level assistant in our department. He was returning every year to teach medical students and residents pathophysiologic mechanisms, clinical picture, and therapies of heart diseases. I risked to be legally responsible for this misconduct. In the end, everything turned out alright. Yiannis returned as a trained cardiologist. Due to his didactic and clinical capabilities, he reached the post of cardiology professor.

What are the points of these stories? Certainly not to accuse anyone of improper behavior. Quite the opposite. I simply want to point out that, in Greece, legal formalities are the scourge of public administration. Anyone in charge of a public organization in our country does not have the same flexibility as his colleagues in Northern Europe or North America. This is because there exists, in these countries, a fundamental atmosphere of trust between the various parties—common sense—even when differences arise on how to proceed. Here everything is reduced to a legal matter, there is no common sense, and there is no well-intentioned disposition that makes a group work together. The rigid legal framework externally imposed on universities, in combination with personal disputes and a lack of trust that chronically undermine our collective mentality, results in the creation of administrative dead ends that on occasion are resolved—tragicomically—by technically illegal actions. This is the most crucial difference between our country and Northern Europe and North America: in order to get things done in Greece conscientiously and efficiently, we very often have to sidestep the law. The conclusion: if you are not careful, the administration of public organizations in Greece will entail a good number of risks. If you want a quiet life, you will behave like a soulless bureaucrat. If you want to be of service, you are at risk. If we as a country manage to solve this paradox—to have to break the law in theory in order to govern in practice—then we will have taken a big step forward. I doubt this is likely to happen.

5.3.2 Clashing with Students

The faculty members, along with two student representatives, met at least once a week for a good number of hours.

It was at one meeting of the faculty, I think in early spring, 1980, that I began to realize what was soon to disturb the smooth upward course of our medical school. Dr. Spyros Doxiades, the Minister of Health, with the help of prominent consultants well-informed about the health sector in Greece, had drawn up a law to modernize the National Health System. In brief, the law proposed full-time and exclusive employment for all employees of the National Health System medical centers and hospitals. It also abolished the waiting list to begin medical specialization, and instead required that national examinations be taken to indicate the candidate's level of knowledge. Based on his or her performance in the exams, the time of specialization would be determined. In other words, the law promoted the concept of merit, which of course faced opposition from those people who would lose their privileges. Doxiades was not a member of the party in power at the time. So, his opposition was both from the left- and the right-wing parties. I studied the law and supported it wholeheartedly.

At that meeting of the medical school faculty, I analyzed all the positive elements in the law. I believe that my recommendations were convincing and that most of my colleagues agreed with my viewpoint. The voting began, to approve or reject publically the law in question, and suddenly, when more than half of the faculty members had already voted in favor of the law, a group of students broke into the meeting hall and demanded that we interrupt our meeting without expressing our opinion on the proposed law. I reacted vigorously. The dean of the medical school, Professor Orestes Tsolas, stood there dumbfounded, like a block of ice.

I kept imploring them not to stop the meeting. Then I spoke to the students. I explained to them that their tactics were violating democratic principles. I told them that their behavior was not suited to that of a future doctor. But my words fell on deaf ears. Then, speaking directly to the dean, with pandemonium breaking loose all around us, I urged him to call the police in order to restore order. As soon as they heard the word "police", the students became even more aggressive and almost violently chased us out of the medical school meeting hall.

The next morning, I went to the Kamperio Cultural Center to teach my course. There were large posters adorning the entrance: "Today Moutsopoulos called the police. Tomorrow he will bring in the tanks," they proclaimed. Again, I paid no attention and began my class. I remember that on that particular day I was teaching a class on the pathogenesis of heart failure. The students were listening attentively to what I had to say. They were feverishly taking notes. All of a sudden, the door of the hall burst open and a swarm of students barged into the room. They impertinently demanded to talk things over. I told them that class hours were not the time for talking anything over. I asked them to leave the room so I could continue my class. I might as well have been talking to the wall. After repeated entreaties for them to leave that went completely unheeded, I was forced to collect my slides and abandon the lecture hall. I made a written report to the rector of the university and the dean of the medical school, concerning the events that had taken place, and concluded the report as follows: "If you cannot assure me a safe and peaceful atmosphere during my classes, I will discontinue them until this simple and reasonable demand is met." The time I was spending treating my patients, ordering new and essential equipment for the clinical department (electrocardiographs, respirators, medicine trolleys with all the necessary instruments for cardiac resuscitation), taking part in the medical school administration, teaching residents based on the patients' problems and showing students how to take a detailed medical history and perform a complete physical examination left me little free time. After two or three weeks of discontinuing my classes in the amphitheater, the student syndicalists asked to see me. Our meeting made it clear to them that I was not fooling around. They realized that I had no inclination to accede to their irrational demands. They asked me to make a public apology. I explained to them that I had no desire to work in a university where fascist tactics prevailed, nor would I be subject to their ridiculous requests. In the end, we agreed that classes would be conducted under civilized conditions. They accepted this and after that everything was fine.

Time rolled along with the intensive rhythms of hard work. Our department continued to improve in offering top-notch medical care to patients. The number of patients we had in the autoimmune rheumatic disease clinic was rising exponentially. Through word of mouth, our clinic had become known throughout Greece. We were consulted by patients from all over the country.

5.3.3 Formalities that Discourage Physician Repatriation

The doctoral degree was, and still is, a necessary qualification for a physician to become a candidate for a faculty position in Greek medical schools. If a candidate for a faculty position does not have this degree, things like superior clinical skills, originality and depth of research work, and dedication to teaching students and physicians, are not considered.

In countries of the West, the doctoral degree is not a necessary qualification for application for a faculty position, or promotion to a higher academic post. Therefore, many experienced Greek physicians who were educated in countries of the West do not have doctoral degrees. The lack of a degree has discouraged many Diaspora physicians, with state-of-the-art medical training and internationally recognized research work, from applying for an academic position in our country.

Upon assuming my professorship in Ioannina, I set a goal for myself: to help any experienced scientists who wanted to repatriate but did not have the coveted Ph.D. Many physicians, who, with my support, received doctoral degrees from the Ioannina University Medical School by submitting the research they had done in laboratories abroad, are serving today in medical schools throughout our country.

It is not my purpose to discuss here who those academics are. I will share with you, however, the reactions caused by these efforts of mine in the spring of 1981. Let me describe the tragicomic events that occurred during the public defense of the doctoral thesis of Vasilis Papadimitriou. Today Vasilis is professor of internal medicine and cardiology at the Georgetown University Medical School, in Washington, D.C.

The question Vasilis was trying to answer through his research studies was why a pregnant woman does not reject an embryo, whose cells contain antigens from its father that are foreign to the mother's body. Physiologically speaking, the mother's immune system should fight them as foreign invaders and reject the embryo from her body. His studies showed that the hormone secreted by the placenta, that is, chorionic gonadotropin, inhibits the mother's immunological reactions against the foreign embryo antigens, so that the embryo is not rejected. The findings of this study were pioneering and could be applied by extension to deterring the rejection of an organ as a foreign body in patients who had undergone transplants.

The day of the public examination arrived. At that time, doctoral theses were evaluated by the entire body of senior faculty members of the medical school. Many of these professors, because of their specialties, could not understand the methodology and the results of Vasilis experiments, or their importance to medical science and their originality. Vasilis, excellently prepared, presented the rationale behind his research, the results of this research, and its possible application for transplants.

I believed that his doctoral degree would be granted with high commendation by the full body of professors. I was shocked when one of my colleagues declared that the dissertation could not be accepted by the medical school. Why? Because it did not state on its cover that the dissertation originated in the department of Internal Medicine of the Ioannina University Medical School, but said that it originated in the immunology laboratory of the National Cancer Institute in America, and also because it said "Bethesda, 1981" on the cover and not "Ioannina, 1981."

These formal omissions were not the true cause of the professor's proposal for the Ioannina University Medical School to reject the thesis. His objections stemmed from his belief that the work on which a doctoral dissertation was based should have been carried out in the Ioannina University Medical School. Anything modern and foreign appeared to frighten him. The quality and the merits of the dissertation did not interest him.

I tried through a series of arguments to convince him that we should in no way encourage young physicians to supply inexact information, not even on the cover of a thesis. If we encourage them to lie, who will prevent them from lying about the methods they use or how the results of their research were obtained? My colleague would hear none of it, however. He insisted that the dissertation could not be accepted by the Ioannina University Medical School.

After an interminable discussion, I accepted a compromise: the cover would mention the laboratory and the city where the work for the dissertation was carried out, as well as the department that approved and brought the dissertation to a vote, and also the city in which the department had its seat, in this case, Ioannina.

After many hours of discussion, Vasilis finally received the long-desired approval of his thesis. But in order to be sworn in as a Ph.D., the poor man had to stay in Ioannina and have a new cover made for his thesis.

It had been Vasilis dream and wish, after finishing his training abroad, to return to Greece and offer his services to patients and his knowledge to students and younger colleagues. The negative experience he had at the defense of his thesis made him reconsider his dream to return to his country. In the end, he decided not to accept the position offered to him by the University of Ioannina and he stayed permanently in America, where he continued his fruitful academic career in cardiology.

5.3.4 Deflecting Unfounded Accusations

It was the beginning of 1981. On the other end of the telephone line was Dr. Dimitris Stroumpoulis, president of the Greek Rheumatology Society, an admiral in the Navy and director of the Athens Naval Hospital, an exceptionally courteous, low-key colleague. We had met in November of 1980 at the Pan-Hellenic Conference of Rheumatology, over which he was presiding. He had invited me to deliver the plenary lecture. I had talked about the immunogenetic basis of autoimmune diseases. With extraordinary tact, he explained to me what he wanted: "The director of the internal medicine department at our hospital, Dr. Antonis Perperas, is an unusually well-trained and cooperative colleague. He did subspecialty studies in the U.K. for two years on diseases of the liver. Although his published research work is quite extensive, your colleagues at the Athens University Medical School will not allow him to submit his research work for consideration for the title of docent. In our profession, rivalries are widespread. Would it be possible for you to meet with him, to form an opinion on his professional achievements and, if you find his work to be up to your standards, could you please support his candidacy at your medical school?".

I had set myself a goal in my professional life to help promote, as much as I could, colleagues who were successful as clinicians and had taken serious steps to acquire new medical knowledge. Based on these criteria, I had helped other worthy colleagues to acquire the title of docent from the Ioannina University Medical School. I agreed to examine the work of the colleague, suggested by the president of the Rheumatology Society. I met with the candidate, I read his papers, and I evaluated his contribution to medical research. He was studying antibodies against a specific lipoprotein of the liver in the blood of patients suffering from virus-induced hepatitis. I found his work satisfactory. So I gave him the green light to apply for the title of docent at our school.

I don't remember how much time went by following my one and only meeting with the candidate. The candidacy of Dr. Perperas came up for approval at the faculty meeting of the medical school. At that meeting, I realized that there was an uneasiness in the air. The Dean of the Medical School, Orestes Tsolas, was having a lively discussion with the representative of the junior faculty, while a group of colleagues had gathered around them to follow their discussion. Soon afterward the meeting began. The subject was brought up of selecting a professor to preside over the evaluation of Dr. Perperas qualifications. The representative of the junior faculty, an attending physician from the Department of Surgery, but above all an experienced syndicalist, solemnly submitted to the faculty body a written accusation against the candidate. In truth, I was alarmed.

I asked to see the accusation. It was an anonymous piece of libel. In brief, the accusation said that "the candidate in question was a collaborator with the colonels' Junta." And it continued by saying that he had found a sympathizer in me, and that because of our shared ideals I was supporting his candidacy. Rather than reveal their names, our small-minded accusers signed "Naval physicians who have learned to wait."

As soon as I read the accusation I calmed down. "A clear sky fears no lightning," I thought. I marveled at the lengths malicious and jealous people will go to. What an imagination people must have to write such inaccurate nonsense. I had no idea what the social or political beliefs of the candidate were. What's more, I have never been influenced by the extracurricular behavior of a candidate except in the case of prosecution for a crime.

I told the faculty body who it was that had recommended the candidate to me, and also that I had only met him once. I stated that I had no social, family, or other relationship with him. I had evaluated, as I always did, the candidate's work, and because I felt that he fulfilled the criteria for the title of docent, I encouraged him to declare his candidacy. I asked two things from the electoral body: first, not to enter the accusation in the records, because I would conclude that the school accepted the accusation and I would press legal charges against the colleague who submitted the anonymous accusation, and also against the administration of the school for spreading and accepting blatant lies concerning my person. And second, I suggested the discussion about the candidate be postponed and that a colleague be appointed to investigate and form an opinion as to whether the charges were true or false.

The colleague who accepted to investigate the charges found nothing incriminating either concerning the candidate or the professor supporting him, meaning me. The procedure for electing him docent continued. The investigation of those charges, however, lengthened the time normally needed to complete the process of awarding the candidate the title of docent. In the end, after the charges were proved false and baseless, the Ioannina University Medical School unanimously granted Mr. Perperas the title of docent of internal medicine. I was left, however, with a bad taste from those anonymous, false accusations, and deep disappointment in the face of the animosity and cowardice of certain individuals.

5.4 Serving as an Elector for New Professors

From the time that I took up the position of professor and chairman of the department of Internal Medicine at the Ioannina University Medical School, I could barely catch my breath with all the obligations I had, each more demanding than the last: treating patients, teaching the students, organizing the department, hiring staff, organizing a research laboratory and giving invited talks at medical schools in other cities in Greece as well as at European or international conferences. Above and beyond all these duties, a full professor had one more academic obligation: participation in the electoral body to choose full or non-tenured professors. The election of new professors determines the future and the direction of our school, that is, whether it will offer high-level education to medical students and physicians in specialty training, provide contemporary medical services to patients, and generate new and innovative medical knowledge. The majority of professors serving as electors were Greeks with a successful academic career either in Europe or the U.S. and relatively untainted by the Greek horse-trading mentality. Discussions were infused with a passion for excellence. Most of us wanted to attract individuals who would serve a dual purpose: the cultivation of excellent physicians but also of pioneering researchers. We wanted our school to be a model academic center for our country. Of course, there were exceptions. "We should support candidates from Ioannina for professorship," several electors hesitantly but insistently whispered. They believed that "locals" would offer more to patient care and to medical education, because they would be permanent residents of Ioannina and not traveling professors only intermittently visiting our city. The electors with this belief were not especially interested in whether the candidates had outstanding academic qualifications.

Most of the professors studied the candidates' curricula vitae carefully, they tried to gather information about their work and their daily lives; they spent a lot of time and placed great importance on a meticulous, almost painstaking, I would say, interview with the candidates. The fact that Epirus was so far from Athens, as well as the inadequate hotel and technical infrastructure of the hospital, discouraged many physicians with excellent academic qualifications from declaring their candidacies. To be honest, only very few had the inclination, the passion, and the self-sacrifice, as it were, to leave behind their comfortable lifestyles abroad, or in the large urban centers in Greece to move to a small provincial town. Many were disturbed by the lack of first-rate private schools for their children; others were bothered by the difficulty of finding work for their spouses.

Quite a few Chairs were vacant. Soon the Chairs of orthopedic surgery, ENT, and ophthalmology were filled. Dermatology and psychiatry, neurology, neurosurgery and cardiovascular surgery were vacant.

One interview in particular of a candidate having roots from Ioannina and seeking for the Chair of neurology has remained very clear in my memory, as though it happened yesterday. I was in my office at the hospital. The morning report of the residents on new admissions and the progress of inpatients in our ward had just finished. I was getting ready for my morning patient rounds. Suddenly, the phone rang. At the other end of the line, I heard the familiar voice of the professor of surgery in our medical school.

"I've got So-and-So here in my office, an esteemed compatriot and one of the best neurologists in Greece. He wants to meet you. I think it would be a great idea if we could elect him to the Chair of neurology," he said, and as his parting shot: "I'm sending him over." He was insistent and I had no time to react.

The candidate showed up at my office soon afterward. His whole demeanor was clearly arrogant, with his spine arched forward, and an ironic and superior expression on his face. He looked down on you. I stood and greeted him. From the beginning of our meeting, he was visibly annoyed. It seems he couldn't accept the fact that a former student of his was now his elector. He seemed not to know or accept that age had nothing to do with academic qualifications. I had studied his curriculum vitae thoroughly. He served for many years at the Athens University Medical School. He had the reputation of being a very good clinician. But he was completely indifferent to researching anything new. His publications were skimpy, limited only to the presentation of interesting medical cases. His post-graduate training abroad had lasted only six months. On his second try, he managed to be elected docent at the Athens University Medical School. In spite of his poor academic profile, it was obvious that he thought quite highly of himself. It is not uncommon for individuals who have not worked at prominent centers abroad, where everyone's activities are evaluated, to create a self-image that does not correspond to reality. As the Cretan adage goes: "The long-necked rooster proudly crows, sees not his faults, and blames his foes."

In an effort to form an objective opinion about the candidate, I tried through our conversation to uncover qualities that may not have been apparent from his curriculum vitae. I asked him what his plans were, in the event that he was elected, for the future of neurology at our medical school. "I will tell you that when I am elected," he answered in an angry tone of voice. Calmly, I continued my inquiry.

"You have an important position in the oldest medical school in the country. What made you want to be a candidate for our medical school?" His answer was completely unexpected. "I do whatever I feel like."

Our meeting finished a few minutes later. He sprang out of his chair and left my office without saying good-bye. Fortunately, the electoral body did not elect him. In turn, an excellent clinician and researcher was elected. He was working as a high-ranking member of the most prominent research institute in the world. We were hoping that his presence and performance at our school would upgrade the field of neurology in our country. When he arrived with his wife to assume his post, instead of starting work, he resigned from his position as professor. And do you know why? Because his wife couldn't find department stores in Ioannina that met her standards. Most probably, this was an excuse. We were searching for excellence, but we came up with nothing.

We encountered a similar problem with the election of another professor of neurosurgery. Two specialists had applied for this Chair. One was educated in the U.K. and worked in the States, and the other was a military physician working in the Veterans Administration Hospital, in Athens. Along with others, I supported the colleague from the West for the Chair. Extremely busy with the obligations of my department, I neglected to do the obvious, to simply ask the candidate's superiors in the U.S. for details on his performance as clinician, teacher, and researcher. The neurosurgeon from abroad was elected and soon took over the directorship of the department. With the help of a powerful local politician, the neurosurgery ward of the hospital was transformed into a luxurious set-up resembling a five-star hotel. To enter the ward an electronic code was required. In that way, the professor's secretary had complete control of all individuals entering the ward. The excuse for these security measures was that they helped avoid crowding and thus prevented post-operative patients from contracting infections. But, in fact, this security measure had another goal, which was to screen those entering the ward. This became apparent through the actions of a clever immigrant, whose wife was waiting to have surgery. The poor man asked to see the professor in order to enquire about the severity of his wife's condition, the type of therapy she would receive, and her long-term prognosis. Using complicated medical terms, the professor confused rather than enlightened the immigrant. In the end, he told him in no uncertain terms that the operation he was about to perform on his wife would be very modern and very expensive. "How much?", the immigrant whispered. Shamelessly, the professor answered: "for you only, it will be x thousands of drachmas." That poor immigrant proved to be smarter than the professor. He went to police headquarters and reported the discussion he had with the professor. The police officer marked the money the professor had demanded from the immigrant, and accompanied him to the professor's office. What followed was that the professor was led out of his office handcuffed and taken to the police. The University Senate, without delay, fired him from his post as professor.

5.5 Life Goes On

In the summer of 1980, I went back to America. My position was activated again. In spite of the hard work there, at the NIH I never felt the emotional exhaustion that I found so distressing in Ioannina when it came to getting even the simplest little thing done. I enjoyed getting back to research at the NIH. Using a high-resolution electrophoretic method developed by Nikos Papadopoulos, we found that patients with Sjögren's syndrome, although they had not yet developed a lymphoid malignancy, had in their bloodstream products of monoclonal B-lymphocytes, denoting a pre-malignant condition. In other words, we had found a way to pinpoint patients who were susceptible to the progression of their disease from benign to malignant. This study was published in *The Journal of Immunology*.

Back in Ioannina, our second academic year (1980–81) brought new and excellently trained faculty members to our department. One of the positions, that of a lecturer, was filled by Stavros Constantopoulos, a pulmonologist trained in America who had been my classmate at the Athens University Medical School. He was already serving at the Athens University Medical School. He was having a lot of problems with the professor holding the Chair there, so he preferred to come and work with us.

The greatest gift of all to our department was the presence of Professor Dimitris Emmanuel from the University of Chicago Medical School. He came to our department on a one-year sabbatical leave. He was an exceptional teacher and researcher, polite, easy to work with, with flawless medical ethics and an incomparable desire to serve others. He was the perfect example of what an academician should be, which was extremely useful during the early years of our medical school. Together we authored the book *Basic Principles of Pathophysiology*. We worked on the various chapters of the book together, along with an additional twenty colleagues from various medical schools around the country. The book was used in other medical schools as a textbook for many years.

When Dimitris' sabbatical year was coming to an end, a position opened up for director of the internal medicine department at the Hatzicostas Hospital. It was a great opportunity to keep this exceptional physician, teacher, and researcher in Ioannina. Dimitris and his family wanted very much to stay in Ioannina. The academic and social atmosphere suited them. He declared his candidacy. We were sure that no other candidate would have the qualifications of Professor Emmanuel. We were both very anxious to work together. Our personalities were very compatible. Our long-term plans were to transform the government internal medicine department into a second university internal medicine department. But alas! The position was filled by a candidate favored by the party in power at the time, a physician without graduate studies, with no teaching experience, with no idea at all what research was all about, and with dubious medical ethics. We made a big fuss through articles in the newspapers. It was all so blatantly unfair. The Minister of Health at the time, Dr. Paraskevas Avgerinos, was upset. He called Dimitris to Athens and urged him to become a candidate for the position of director of nephrology, which had just been announced at the Laïko General Hospital, in Athens. Dimitris did this and was appointed director with high commendation. In the end, the students of the medical school of the University of Ioannina, the residents, the attending physicians, and the patients were deprived of an excellent physician, teacher, researcher, and an unusual human being with great sensitivity and selflessness in treating his patients.

Starting that year, other new faculty members were included in the department's voluntary teaching staff. Their contribution was fundamental. One was Giorgos Chrousos, an endocrinologist from the NIH in America, and another was Yiannis Daniilidis, an internist-gastroenterologist also trained in America. Yiannis and I first met in 1973–1974. I was a resident and he was an intern at the Veterans Administration Hospital, in Washington, D.C. I was impressed by his extensive medical knowledge, his industriousness, and his serious personality. Our paths diverged when I went to San Francisco and he to Texas. We met again in Greece. He was director of the Department of Gastroenterology at Athens General State Hospital. Because of his work in research, the medical school of the University of Ioannina awarded him the title of docent. And so, little by little, we were able to cover more and more of the major sections of internal medicine in our department.

The lack of space was becoming increasingly pressing day by day. The room for the night-shift doctors was used during the day as a pulmonology and bronchoscopy outpatient clinic. The hospital did not have a bronchoscope. Stavros Constantopoulos generously performed bronchoscopies on patients with his own personal broncho- scope. The internal medicine department, instead of an old age home or a sick patients' depot, was now beginning to resemble a tertiary medical care facility.

The outpatient clinic for autoimmune rheumatic diseases reminded us every day of the need to create a diagnostic immunology laboratory. In order to diagnose and provide a prognosis for a patient with autoimmune rheumatic disease and to monitor the response to therapeutic intervention, we needed to have at our disposal different immune parameters, such as autoantibodies against various self-antigens, the level of acute-phase proteins, as well as complement proteins, in a patient's blood. The university microbiology laboratory had no inclination to help us. We had to develop our own immunology laboratory.

A space was found for us to set up the laboratory: two rooms in the old Hatzicostas Hospital, next to the morgue, where as a student I had my first lessons in research. The top floor of the old Hatzicostas Hospital functioned as a two-year nursing school. The technical staff of the hospital made the necessary changes: installing workbenches, painting, and upgrading the overall appearance of the space. With donations from grateful patients, the first essential instruments were purchased.

The first volunteer assistants were two fourth-year medical students, Panayotis Vlachoyiannopoulos and Athanasios Tzioufas, and a third-year medical student, Menelaus Manoussakis, all with a fervid interest in learning, all very cooperative and eager to offer their services. With the help of the lecturer, Anestis Mavridis, from the department of Microbiology, they quickly set up the first essential immunology tests. Today, the first two of these talented and dedicated students, after important research and work toward understanding the pathogenesis of autoimmune rheumatic diseases, are professors at the Athens University Medical School, both internationally recognized for their contributions to research. Anestis Mavridis is an emeritus professor of microbiology at the Ioannina University Medical School.

The newly established immunology laboratory, aside from its contribution to everyday diagnostics, rapidly became a hub for generating new medical knowledge. Based on the specifics of our space, our instruments, and the money we had available, I had to decide in which area to focus our research on understanding the pathogenesis of autoimmune diseases. In America, I had enjoyed studying human cellular immunology and the mice models of autoimmune diseases. That type of research requires specific facilities, a lot of money and specialized instruments, and personnel. So, back in Ioannina, I decided to turn our research interests toward antibody-mediated autoimmunity, that is, the study of autoantibodies and other immune-functioning proteins. Fotini Skopouli, a resident at that time, was sent to Bath Medical Center, in England, to work in the immunology laboratory for three months. She learned to set up the methodology for the detection of autoantibodies, which she brought back to our laboratory. In order to test for autoantibodies in patients' sera, the presence of antigens against which the autoantibodies react is necessary. These antigens are acquired from the bovine thymus or spleen. The Ioannina slaughterhouse was very close to our laboratory, so we had plenty of beef tissue to use for preparing the autoantigens we needed, and at no cost.

The outpatient clinic for patients with autoimmune rheumatic diseases operated in the narrow confines of my office. It was organized perfectly by Tereza Papadopoulou and two young physicians, Alekos Drossos and Fotini Skopouli (Photo 5.2). Neither of these two physicians allowed themselves any time for self-indulgence. And, so, with their unbounded appetite for acquiring new knowledge, their diligence in keeping up-to-date with the latest developments in our field, and with Alekos organizational skills and Fotini's meticulous and thorough work, the outpatient clinic of autoimmune rheumatic diseases was now operating at a level equal to, or even higher than that in countries with advanced healthcare systems. Today, Alekos is emeritus professor of rheumatology at the Ioannina University Medical School, and Fotini is

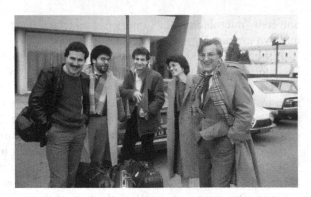

Photo 5.2 From left to right: Alexandros Drossos, Athanasios Tzioufas, Menelaus Manoussakis, Fotini Skopouli and author

emerita professor of internal medicine and immunology at Harokopio University, in Athens.

We had created special medical records for our patients to follow them up. Thus, at any given moment we had at our disposal the clinical picture, the applied therapies, and the medical progress of every patient. The information in the patients' records was a valuable source of material for our clinical and laboratory research studies. We were consulted by patients with very serious autoimmune rheumatic diseases. Every patient, who believed we had solved his problems, would bring us another patient with similar problems. That is how things work in our country. The patients send other patients to the specialist. So, patients found their way to Ioannina because of the fast-spreading reputation of our center for autoimmune rheumatic diseases. Another source of patient referrals to our department was from colleagues abroad who saw patients from Greece.

In view of the continuous training program we implemented, the increased number of patients our center was attracting and the substantial number of high-quality faculty members we had appointed to the university internal medicine department, the Ministry of Health designated our department as a center able to provide training in internal medicine and rheumatology to young physicians seeking to be specialized. The number of residents in the internal medicine department increased from five to ten, and four new positions were instituted for trainees in rheumatology.

5.6   Administrative Obstacles

The relatively rapid increase in trainees in our department, the doubling of the number of third- and fourth-year students in the medical school who were being trained in the hospital, and a large number of physicians serving in other departments of the hospital who came voluntarily to attend our post-graduate training program, made the chairman's office inadequate as a room to teach in. I asked the hospital administration to convert one of the patient wards into a classroom and a library. The chief administrator, although a physician himself, was not able to see the value of such a classroom. He preferred to have more rooms for treating patients. In spite of the administration's reaction, with the help of the nurses, I emptied the six-patient ward. With the assistance of a local businessman, Mr. Petsios, the walls of the classroom were covered with metal shelves and the classroom was filled up with desks, bought with a donation from a pharmaceutical company. The small classroom-and-library was now quite presentable. This news reached the administration. The chief administrator sent me a notice asking me to account for my actions. Instead I called him and gave him a piece of my mind. I told him that if he continued fighting the medical school I would report it to the office of the district attorney and also inform the press. Most likely my threats, or perhaps the explanations I gave him—who knows?—stopped him. From that time on and until we moved, many years later, to the new University Hospital, that classroom was teeming with life. The shelves were filled with my personal books and journals, which I had collected over many years, brought back with me from America, and donated to the hospital for the education of our students and physicians. That classroom also served, during the evening shifts, as an office for the residents of our department. The post-graduate sessions held in the newly developed classroom were very popular. Students, residents, and staff members were all anxious to find a place and attend the educational seminars.

5.7 Back to Work

The remainder of that academic year went by without further upheavals. Together with the newly appointed faculty members of our department, we started giving courses to private physicians in Ioannina. We also gave seminars, when invited, to different medical associations, and in other cities.

The first seminar we gave was on the clinical expression, differential diagnosis, diagnosis, and treatment of systemic lupus erythematosus, the main example of autoimmune rheumatic disease. We gave seminars to colleagues in other cities in our region, such as Larissa, Arta, and Corfu. We were invited to give a seminar by the Medical & Surgical Society of Corfu, the oldest medical association in our country. In one session we discussed inflammatory arthritis, and in another viral-induced hepatitis. We had also taken the fourth-year medical students there with us. Our seminar was very well received. The president of the Medical & Surgical Society of Corfu, Dr. Yiannis Moraitis, was very enthusiastic. He gave me as a keepsake the first bell ever used by the president of the society to open a session—a collector's item over one hundred years old. It has had a prominent place on my desk ever since.

During that academic year, I received a scholarship from the British Council to visit rheumatology and immunology departments in the U.K. at such places as Guy's Hospital, Hammersmith Hospital, Middlesex Hospital, the Kennedy Institute of Rheumatology, and the Bath Hospital Center. There, I gave lectures based on my research findings and discussed their research programs. I came to realize through these visits that the U.K. was scientifically far behind the U.S, and to my surprise I learnt that, even well-known researchers of inflammatory diseases didn't recognize

Photo 5.3 Editors of
Clinical and Experimental
Rheumatology. From left to
right: Paul Philips, author,
Stefano Bombardieri,
Graham Hughes, Barbara
Ansell, Giampiero Passero,
Raffaele Numo and
secretaries, Luisa
Marconcini and Lisa Chien

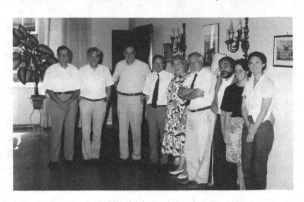

the entity Sjögren's syndrome, a relatively common disorder with unique clinic-laboratory picture. That experience gave me hope that I would be able to succeed in creating a model and pioneering research center in my own country. Nowadays, over 40 years later, every European country has a center studying this syndrome.

My educational activities in research that year also extended to Europe. Professor Gabriel Panayi from Guy's Hospital Medical School and I organized a yearly meeting of colleagues from European countries, called the "European Workshop for Rheumatology Research." Over a two-day period, the research findings of different groups from all over Europe were presented and discussed. That meeting was and still is the top-ranking European scientific event in our field.

My colleagues, Professors Stefano Bombardieri, from Pisa, Italy, Paul Phillips, from Syracuse, NY, and Graham Hughes, from London, and I created a new medical journal, *Clinical and Experimental Rheumatology* (Photo 5.3).

Summer came and it was time for me to go back to America to continue my research. Beginning that summer, and for all the summers that followed, I no longer went alone to America. I had announced to the medical students that I would be delighted if anyone wanted to accompany me and discover the beauty of research at the largest biomedical center in the world, the NIH. Three students came with me in the summer of 1981. They were Dimitris Boumpas, Sakis Koukoumpis, and Konstantinos Kolios. I had arranged free room and board for them at the hostel of St. George's Church, so that their families would only have to pay their airfare and give them pocket money for their day-to-day living expenses. Dimitris worked with me at the immunology laboratory. It has been many years since 1981. I don't remember where the other two students worked. At the end of two months, they had all gained medical knowledge, their English was much improved, and their social contacts had enhanced their personalities.

Upon our return to Ioannina from our summer research work in America, there was a lot of work waiting for me in terms of improving the medical and educational activities of our department, including hiring new specialists in various sections of internal medicine who would help upgrade patients' care and the department's pre- and post-graduate educational program.

5.8 The University Framework Law: Radical Change

The elections of 1981 brought "the people to power." The Pan-Hellenic Socialist Movement, known by its Greek initials as PASOK, won by a large majority and became the new government. The pre-election promises for changes to the health sector, the universities and the social infrastructure were implemented one after the other. You could feel that change was in the wind.

The people in charge at the Ministry of Education, with their advisors, attending physicians under the thumb of their boss professor, all high on the new catchword "change," set themselves the goal of abolishing the university Chair. They believed, and rightly so, that it had to be done away with. Their purpose was to curb the absolute power of the full professor. Undoubtedly, all those who undertook to design the new laws were not devoid of good intentions. But many of them did not have academic qualifications, and unfortunately had not served in a functional university, in an advanced country. They copied legal statutes from English-speaking countries without including, however, important provisions such as those regarding merit.

When I read the "Framework Law," as they liked to call law 1268/1982, I thought at first that I was in familiar territory. I was the first one who had supported, without a framework law, the idea of sections within departments of the Ioannina University of Medical School, slowly and steadily abolishing the outdated Chair. I soon realized, however, that the new law included traps that, instead of improving the administration and the functioning of the university, could gradually lead to its decline.

The first incorrect provision of the new law was that it promoted the already employed members of the junior faculty, without any evaluation, to various professorial positions. Those devising the law forgot, or did not take into account, the fact that those serving under the all-powerful full professor were hired in his image. His co-workers were, for the most part, individuals with modest academic potential and often with weak characters that could put up with the "despot." The new law, instead of requiring the evaluation of those already serving, simply re-named doctoral degree-holding teaching assistants "lecturers," and duly elected docents were re-named "assistant professors." Docents by appointment were now called "associate professors," and full professors were now just "professors." The only ones who were evaluated in order to acquire a new professorial position were the expert consultants who, according to their achievements, could become either assistant or associate professors. Without delay, the junior faculty members of the medical schools created unions, whose goal was to promote their own interests as civil servants, not the interests of the university and, by extension, of society at large. And they did this not with ill intentions, but because that is what they knew how to do, and that is what they did. They never had the opportunity to experience the beauty of a good university. They never saw nor did they wish to learn how academic centers of excellence were created.

The second great crime, which began and continued with the implementation of the new law, was that the administrative officials of the university—department and laboratory directors, school presidents, deans, and rectors—would be elected by their subordinates, that is, by the same people they would eventually be evaluating for promotion to higher-ranking positions. This was conducive to the exchange of favors and fostered corruption. So those wanting to govern the university, who were responsible for its efficient functioning, would make deals with their younger colleagues, turn a blind eye to their academic improprieties, indulge the unionists and satisfy their every irrational demand to sabotage the creation of innovative new knowledge. In this way, the highest-ranking administrative positions in the university were filled by elected individuals with limited academic qualifications, and with no significant presence in the international academic community. This sad state of affairs is beautifully outlined in a book written by Theodoros Lazaridis. So, when the leaders of the academic community are lacking in qualifications, why should anyone believe or hope that the other members of the university community will have academic qualifications? Entangled interests, the trading of favors and nepotism in general have turned our universities into rear-guard laggards far from the front lines of international scientific developments.

The above crimes were carried out with the participation of students in the election of administrative officials. The new young scholars, instead of involving themselves in the promotion of knowledge, free thinking, and excellence, became pawns in a favor-trading game played out between their teachers, union bigwigs, and vote-seeking politicians.

The third Greek innovation ushered in by the new law was the preferential treatment of already serving members on the teaching and research faculty when it came to promotions, to the detriment of the candidates who were not in the faculty but had better academic qualifications. Because of this, junior faculty members who had been at the same level for twenty years managed, within a few years, to become professors.

This phenomenon can aptly be described as "inbreeding." It is well known that inbreeding, in nature, meaning interbreeding of closely related individuals, will quite probably lead to genetic defects in their offspring. This is what happened to our universities.

During the period when the military Junta ruled Greece (1967–1974), the Security Police had free rein in the universities. They kept students and teachers under strict surveillance. They would arrest democratically thinking and speaking members of the university community and subject them to exhaustive interrogations using psychological and physical abuse. With the restoration of democracy in the country, a provision was included in this new law that was specifically designed to protect protesting students from the police. It defined the university as an "asylum," meaning that a university is an academic sanctuary where everyone can express ideas freely. The police could no longer enter university premises, unless they were summoned by the university senate to prevent a criminal act, or arrest someone committing an illegal act. But the unions and activists on the university teaching and research staff managed, due to the inability of those in power to run the university and the state, to debase and take advantage of the concept of asylum. And so, at the slightest provocation, the university would be occupied by groups of students and others, who barred students and members of the teaching and research staff from entering the university.

Course hours were lost, graduate students were prevented from carrying out their experiments, laboratories were destroyed and no one dared to ask that the damaged or stolen items be replaced. The idea of sending those students responsible before a disciplinary council was never even discussed. The high-ranking university administrative officials owe a lot to the students who occupy the university and destroy public property, since they play a significant role in electing those officials to their positions. The people who occupy and dishonor the university are the same people who hold street demonstrations, go on strike, and stop classes for no good reason, without anyone so much as lifting a finger.

5.9   Solving Public Health Problems

Frequent student strikes and sit-ins continued to plague our university. In spite of all this, the internal medicine department was improving day by day.

Clinical and immunologic studies carried out entirely in Ioannina, or in collaboration with research centers abroad, were being published. Not only that, but aside from studies on autoimmune rheumatic diseases, two important public health problems in our area were solved. The first was "Metsovo lung." My and Stavros Constantopoulos interest, in studying this condition, began with chest X-rays of people from Metsovo that made us suspect that the residents of that area were suffering from asbestosis, a lung condition caused by inhalation of asbestos dust (a fibrous-textured incombustible mineral). An unusually large number of people from that same area also developed a rare cancer of the pleura, the membrane covering the lungs, that is, the mesothelioma. We had calculated, based on the number of patients, that residents of the Metsovo area were three hundred times more likely than other Greeks to develop this type of cancer.

Clinical, radiological and pathology studies confirmed that the damage observed in the X-rays was indeed asbestosis. This was most likely not due to workplace exposure to asbestos, seeing as there was no factory in the area producing or using asbestos. It was probably due to breathing in asbestos from the atmosphere.

With the help of the mayor of Metsovo, one Sunday after church, we held a town meeting. All the men, women, and children from Metsovo were there. After we explained the problem and its effect on their health, we asked the residents if they or others in the area were using any unusual substances at home or elsewhere.

A young man, Michalis Tritos, a teacher of religion in the Metsovo High School, solved the puzzle.

"We paint our houses with this material. Could it be asbestos?" He showed us a whitish, compact ball.

The material was sent to a specialized research center in New York. It was, indeed, asbestos. Naturally, we notified the residents of Metsovo and the surrounding villages. The use of that material to paint houses was discontinued. Many years later, the lung X-rays of younger residents of Metsovo did not present the picture of asbestosis.

The second problem occurred in the summer of 1982, when our medical wards were inundated with individuals with a high fever and other symptoms and indications pointing to leptospirosis. The examinations, however, did not confirm that diagnosis.

I discussed this medical problem with a colleague from the Athens University Medical School. He was a specialist in infectious diseases. But he couldn't help me.

I phoned the Disease Control Center in Atlanta, Georgia, in the U.S., and spoke to an expert on hemorrhagic fever. I described the clinical and laboratory picture of the patients. He answered immediately: "It seems that you have in your area an epidemic of Korean hemorrhagic fever affecting the kidneys. This is an infection in humans caused by polluted water from the urine of infected yellow field mice. The specialist in your country for this illness is Professor Antonis Antoniadis at the Thessaloniki University Medical School."

As soon as I received this information, I was relieved. I was increasingly hopeful that we could now solve this unfamiliar public health problem.

I contacted Professor Antonios Antoniadis immediately. From our very first conversation, he was very cooperative. On the next bus out, we sent him blood samples from our patients. All the blood samples were positive for antibodies against the Korean virus. Thus, the cause of this endemic infection was identified. With the help of the agronomic services, the farmers were instructed on how to get rid of these mice in order to protect the health of the inhabitants of the area and the produce from their fields.

5.10   Unexpected Difficulties on a Scientific Trip to Turkey

In the fall of 1982, I received an invitation to visit the Cerrahpaşa University Hospital, in Istanbul, and to deliver the plenary lecture at the annual Turkish Rheumatology Conference. I accepted the invitation without a second thought. I was pleased and very proud. Pleased because I had an opportunity to visit the "Queen of all cities," and proud because colleagues from a not-so-friendly neighboring country, at a time when it was under military rule, were doing me the honor of letting me teach them.

When I landed in Istanbul in May of 1983, I was greeted by a sun-filled day. Waiting for me at the airport was Professor Hasan Yaziçi, an internationally renowned expert on the Adamantiadis-Behçet syndrome, an inflammation of small blood vessels, clinically manifested by aphthous ulcers on the mouth, the genitals, and eye inflammation.

He had been trained in America too. We knew each other through our published scientific work. But it was the first time we met in person. Standing tall and erect, he politely expressed his pleasure that we were finally meeting.

I would be staying in Istanbul for three days. On the first day, I would have a chance to see the sights, the second would be taken up with visiting the University Hospital and giving my talk, and on the third day, I had arranged through the Bishop of Ioannina a visit to the patriarchate and the Ecumenical Patriarch.

I haven't the words to describe the beauty of Istanbul. This has been done by others, moreover, and a lot better than I could do it.

Walking through the streets of the city, I noticed that on every street corner an army tank was stationed. Without thinking, I asked: "Why so much military?".

They looked at me with curiosity. They reminded me in a few well-chosen words that their country was under military rule.

Words are not enough to describe to you the extent of Professor Yazıçı's hospitality. I stayed in a neoclassical building for visiting professors belonging to the university, on the Bosporus, next to a mosque. The room was simple, but with all the necessary amenities for a comfortable stay. From the window of that room you could see the Bosporus and the historic neighborhood of Pera, now called Beyoğlu. Aside from the delicious meals they served us, I had a chance to see the dance of the whirling dervishes for the first time.

At the hospital I was confronted with the same sights as in a Greek hospital: men, women, and children one on top of the other in the outpatient clinics. Wards for treating eight patients were occupied by ten to twelve patients. There were poorly equipped diagnostic laboratories. I am sure that if the visiting professor were a colleague from an economically developed country, he would wonder how innovative medical knowledge was generated in this third-world country. "It's passion and love for research that really counts, not first-world luxuries," I thought. In contrast to the picture of the patient wards, the professors' offices were quite lavish. The furniture was impressive, the bookcases filled with books and journals.

I discussed a good number of medical cases that they described to me, and I gave a talk on the pathogenesis of autoimmune diseases. After a sumptuous meal looking out on the Bosporus, it was time to deliver the plenary address at the National Rheumatology Meeting.

The amphitheater was packed. I presented clinical, immunological, and immunogenetic studies that showed the differences between Greek and Anglo-Saxon patients with rheumatoid arthritis. All of the scientific data I cited came from our collaboration with Professor Gabriel Panayi at Guy's University Hospital in London. This work was published in *Arthritis and Rheumatism*.

While presenting the immunogenetic differences between Greek and English patients, I made a comment in which I jokingly referred to the period of Ottoman rule over Greece: "Why don't you look at the immunogenetic underpinnings of your patients with rheumatoid arthritis?" And I continued: "Maybe our immunogenetic data is similar to yours, seeing as we lived together for four hundred years, so it's possible that our genetic material was interchanged."

I finished my talk and answered the questions that were posed to me. I was pleased with my performance.

As I was stepping down from the podium, two dark-skinned men in rather shabby black suits, with a frown on their faces and glowering eyes, came up to me and, in perfect English, asked me what I meant when I said that our genetic materials had been interchanged for many years. I tried to explain to them that I was joking. They looked at me circumspectly and asked me almost rudely if I could give them a written copy of my talk.

"I can give you the slides," I said, "but I have no written copy of my talk."

The speedy arrival of Professor Yazıçi on the scene helped clear things up. He talked to them, in a loud tone of voice, for quite some time. I watched the expressions on their faces. Their conversation slowly became calmer and they soon left the room. I thought that was the end of the matter.

At dinner, I found a minute to ask Professor Yazıçi who those men were and why they wanted a copy of my talk. From what he told me, I understood that they were Turkish Central Intelligence agents.

The following day, I visited Patriarch Dimitrios with Professor Yazıçi, and his sister. She was a historian and a professor at the university. She had been looking for an opportunity to meet the Patriarch for a long time. We were all impressed by the geniality and mildness of his character and the simplicity of his behavior.

The rest of the visit to Istanbul went by with no further incidents, and with nothing but the most colorful impressions of its natural and architectural sights and the incomparable hospitality of its inhabitants.

The surprise came after I landed at the Hellenic Airport, in Athens. At passport control, the policeman on duty informed me that I had to see his superior officer. In truth, I was quite shaken by this. But I pulled myself together and asked him why.

"There's a problem with your passport," he said, and continued: "Your passport has been stamped by the Turkish-controlled part of Cyprus, which is forbidden on Greek documents."

I was taken aback by this statement. Without realizing it, I stammered:

"That's very strange. I did not visit Turkish-controlled Cyprus, and have only just returned from Istanbul."

My "friends" at the Turkish Intelligence Agency had set me up. It was obvious that they did this because of the joke I made during my talk.

After speaking with his superior, the Greek officer on duty urged me, as soon as I returned to work, to write a report to the Greek State Intelligence Agency listing all the details of my visit to Istanbul. Once I did this, the forbidden stamp in my passport would cease to be valid.

After some time, when Professor Yazıçi and I met again at a conference, he confided in me that he also paid dearly for his visit to the Patriarch. For many months, he was interrogated every afternoon by the Istanbul Security Police. They wanted to know what we had talked about with the Christian leader. Fortunately, there were no further complications. A lovely experience was almost ruined, and all because of a joke.

5.11   Setting Standards for Academic Promotion

At the Ioannina University Medical School, members of the junior faculty who did not have satisfactory academic credentials, or who belonged to political parties began to form unions. For them, the university was a sideline. Their goal was to have a career in politics. In one instance those junior faculty members tried, along with the student representatives of political parties, to impose the upgrading of one of the expert consultants to the rank of associate professor.

The position of expert consultant had been voted into law for the new medical schools. The position was usually given to individuals with qualifications that were superior to those of a lecturer. The colleague in question had done two years of subspecialty studies in gynecological endocrinology abroad. During that time, his research activities were satisfactory, but his overall achievements were far below what the law prescribed for the position of associate professor. His union colleagues believed that if they succeeded in convincing or bullying the electoral body into awarding the position of associate professor to that consultant, then the road would be open for anyone, regardless of qualifications, to be promoted to the highest academic ranks. Here, I must in all fairness mention that the candidate being supported for the position of associate professor by his fellow unionists was better qualified than his department chairman, and he had a scientific profile that showed great promise for the future.

In 1983, I spent the entire summer at the NIH, in America. I wanted to finish up some research projects but, to be perfectly honest, I mainly wanted to decide whether I would return to Greece or stay in America. At this point, the reader may wonder why I was so ambivalent. It was because, on the one hand, I had foreseen the irregularities that the new law would cause in the universities, and, on the other, my relationship with Lambrini, after some rather troubled years, had been broken off. In the end, after much thought, I decided that I should return to Greece and deal with these problems there and then.

I returned to Ioannina the day before the above-mentioned colleague's election was scheduled to take place. It was my habit to go directly from the plane to my office. The university Chairs had administrative offices on the first floor of the newly renovated Georgiou Stavrou building in an area of Ioannina called "Yiali Kafene." The name was left over from the several hundred years that the area was occupied by the Ottoman Turks. On the ground floor of the same building, a long, narrow room had been made into a classroom.

Before I even had time to be briefed on pending matters by my secretaries, the colleague whose promotion was going to be put to a vote the next day appeared in the doorway of my office. He very politely asked if we could meet to discuss his candidacy. We made an appointment late that afternoon. When we met, I tried to get across to him that it was inappropriate for him to be pressuring people to elect him to the rank of associate professor. I urged him instead to apply for the position of assistant professor. Once he was elected, after a reasonable amount of time had passed, he could again go abroad in order to acquire additional clinical and research experience. I don't believe he heard a word I was saying. He smugly assured me that the following day all the professors, except for me, would vote for him as associate professor.

The time for his election arrived. The student representatives and the representatives of the junior faculty seemed ready for battle. They were discussing, in small groups, their strategy, or so I would like to believe, for achieving their goal. The election got underway. The written evaluation of his accomplishments was read by the president of the search committee. It was unequivocally in favor of the candidate. It is common practice in Greek universities for electors who know that a candidate does not have the necessary qualifications to nonetheless write something positive about him. In that way, they stay on good terms with everyone and leave it to the remaining few "crazy" professors to pull the chestnuts out of the fire. This is what happened in the above election.

When it was my turn to speak, I believe I impartially analyzed the strong and weak qualifications of the candidate, and I made the same suggestions to the electoral body as I had to the candidate himself.

Right after me, the representative of the junior faculty took the floor. He was provocative and aggressive. I did not leave his statements unanswered. Pandemonium ensued. There was nasty shouting from all sides. The election procedure was cut short. After a proposal by the student representatives and the representatives of the junior faculty, the Rector's Council began the procedure of sending me before the Disciplinary Council with the charge of "ill-advised academic behavior." For reasons I am unaware of, that procedure was never completed. In the end, the election was never held either, and the candidate followed my suggestion and took two years of sabbatical leave. Upon his return he was elected associate professor, and several years later he was elected professor and director of obstetrics and gynecology at the Thessaly University Medical School.

5.12 Scientific Trips Behind the Iron Curtain

My first professional visit to Moscow was in the late 1970s. I was a member of a U.S. team. The purpose of the visit was to establish medical scientific collaborations with our colleagues from the Union of Soviet Socialist Republics (U.S.S.R.). The head of the team was Dr. John L. Decker, and the other members were Professor Roger William, Dr. Paul Plotz, Professor Eng Tan, and myself. The meetings were held at the Institute of Rheumatology, a part of the U.S.S.R. Academy of Medicine. The head of the institute was Professor Valentina Nassonova, a middle-aged, serious, well-dressed, impressive woman. We met all the institute members in person. They listened to our talks, and we listened to theirs. All the talks presented the major accomplishments of U.S. and U.S.S.R. researchers. The atmosphere was very friendly. After many long hours of meetings, in the evenings, we had superb dinners at the best restaurants, in Moscow. On the third and last day, after the farewell dinner, they took us to the Bolshoi ballet. I can't really say if this visit had any significant results or any significant gains for either side of the curtain.

My second visit to Moscow was in 1983. I was a speaker at the European Rheumatology meeting, which was organized by the USSR Institute of Rheumatology. I stayed in Moscow only for the day I gave the lecture. Then I flew to Vilnius, Lithuania, because I had arranged, while in the USSR, to present the results of our research to the Rheumatology Society of Lithuania. I stayed there for one day as well, because the next day my good friend and enthusiastic researcher of Sjögren's syndrome, Dr.

Vladimir Vassiliev, was going to be married in Red Square. I was to be their best man.

After the formal dinner, I took the train in order to get to Moscow on time. It is difficult to describe my experience on that overnight train trip. I didn't sleep at all. The noise of the train, the loud discussions in the cabin, the periodic crowing of the roosters, and bleating of sheep accompanying the passengers kept me awake. I arrived in Moscow on Saturday noon completely exhausted. There were around ten couples waiting to get married, surrounded by friends and relatives. The number of people around Vladimir and his bride was limited. They sang something from a book and that was the entire marriage ceremony. Vladimir was getting married for the second time. The major problem for the newly married couple was where to make their nest. In Moscow, because it is so highly crowded, if you divorce and leave the apartment where you had been staying with your first wife, it is impossible to find another place in the city. Everything is occupied. Vladimir found an apartment two hours outside Moscow. The distance didn't seem to bother them. They were very happy.

My third and last visit to the USSR was in the middle of 1985. Professor Valentina Nassonova invited all the members of my team researching different aspects of autoimmune rheumatic diseases to visit the Institute of Rheumatology. Visits to the USSR were always enjoyable. The only negative memory was the long lines of people waiting patiently to pass through customs. Even if you were an official invitee, the interrogations you had to go through were the same for everyone.

On this visit, our team consisted of thirteen people (Photo 5.4). Our secretaries also came with us. All expenses were covered by the hosts. We arrived at the Hotel Moscow, located in Red Square and overlooking the river Volga, late in the evening. We asked the colleague who was acting as our guide where to eat supper. He informed us that restaurants in Moscow close at 8:00 p.m. but that small canteens might be open on certain floors of our hotel. Fotini Skopouli, my colleague and also my girlfriend, and I bought a roasted chicken and a bottle of red wine and enjoyed them in our room.

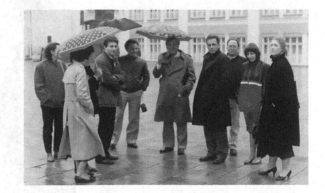

Photo 5.4 The team going to Moscow. From left to right: Fotini Skopouli, Yiotanna Dalavanga, Menelaus Manoussakis, Nikos Pavlidis, author, Nikiforos Angelopoulos, Stavros Constantopoulos and two colleagues from the Rheumatology Institute of the USSR academy

The next morning, after breakfast, a small bus took us to the institute. All the senior members were waiting there with Professor Nassonova, who was obviously in charge (Photo 5.5). Also with her were Professor Gusseva, an expert on scleroderma, Dr. S. Soloviev, an expert on lupus, Dr. Vladimir Vassiliev, an expert on Sjögren's syndrome, Professor A. D. Speransky, the head of the immunology laboratory, and others. Our two-day program was packed with lectures (Photo 5.6) and discussions about future experiments and therapeutic protocols. During this meeting, Professor Nassonova and I arranged for Dr. Vassiliev to work in our lab for three months, supported by a small stipend from the Society for Epirote Studies, an organization that had developed a special research account for donations from grateful patients, business people and others.

Our first dinner took place in the restaurant of the hotel. The food was uninteresting, but we enjoyed the songs of a famous Russian singer. The last dinner

Photo 5.5 Author, Professors Valentina Nassonova and Natalia Gusseva

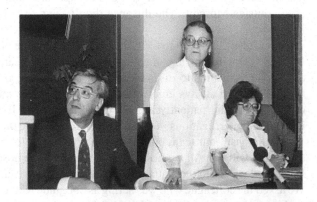

Photo 5.6 Author delivering a lecture

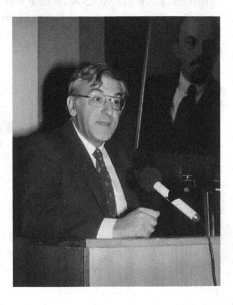

was in a famous restaurant where I had also been invited the first time I visited Moscow. After dinner, they took us to the Bolshoi ballet. As we were leaving the ballet, Vassiliev and Soloviev came over to Fotini and me and invited us to Soloviev's home. We happily accepted their invitation. Without losing any time, they stopped a military vehicle, and after a short conversation we all got in. A short while later we arrived at a well-furnished apartment, where we enjoyed plenty of vodka and relaxing conversation.

At around midnight the phone rang. Dr. Soloviev answered it. Someone wanted to talk to me. I was really surprised. I took the phone from him. On the other end of the line was the colleague who was supposed to be our guide. Like a teacher supervising children on a school excursion, he told me that we were supposed to be in our room. Slightly tipsy, with all that Vodka in my system, I told him that we were much better off where we were than in our room. He insisted that we return to the hotel and informed me that a car was waiting outside the apartment complex to take us there. We didn't have a choice; we had to leave our pleasant companions. While we were leaving Soloviev's apartment, our friends whispered that our guide was an agent appointed by the State Security Commission (KGB) to keep an eye on us.

After a most exciting time, the next morning we returned home to find a lot of work waiting for all of us.

5.13 An Experience in Israel

I hope that the reader won't think that I was prejudiced when I was criticizing our close surveillance by a KGB agent during our visit to Moscow. Such phenomena can happen in democratic states.

Let me share with you my experience during a scientific visit to Israel.

I was invited to an International Hematology meeting to present our work in cryo-globulins, which are proteins-antibodies precipitating in cold temperature; they can be found in the sera of patients with hematopoietic malignancies and autoimmune rheumatic diseases. The meeting took place in Jerusalem. In that trip I was accompanied by my son Thucydides ("Thuk"). It was an opportunity for him to see all the historic sites of the city where three religions coexisted and that, I must confess not in an harmonic way.

We were accommodated in a beautiful hotel in the new city. By the time we arrived in the hotel it was late evening; after a shower and a delightful dinner it was time for us to rest. The following day was free. My lecture was scheduled for the next day. "Thuk", after carefully studying Jerusalem travel guides, was prepared to visit the interesting sites of the old city. Before starting our tour, we had to pay a visit to the mother of a classmate and friend of mine, Suhel Abu Gazales. In fact, our apartments in Athens were on the same condominium. He was a recipient of a scholarship of the Jerusalem Patriarchate, and was also studying Medicine at the Athens University Medical School. His father was relative of the King Hussein, and was serving as the Major of Jerusalem before the city was occupied by the Israelis.

Suhel had a successful rising academic path in the USA. He quickly became a Professor of Emergency Medicine in Tennessee. His book on Emergency Medicine was considered as a classic one. We kept in contact, either when he was visiting Greece or by telephone. I knew that his mother was still living in Jerusalem, while his brother had moved to Amman and was working there as a manager of an international company. After an enjoyable breakfast, we went to a taxi stand. I carefully searched for a Palestinian taxi driver. I identified one without special difficulty. I asked him if he could take us to ex-Major Gazales house. Soon we arrived there and we were ringing the Gonzales' doorbell. An elderly, well-dressed lady, opened the door of the home. I presented myself and introduced "Thuk". She welcomed us like if we were close relatives. She led us to sit in the home's reception room. I described to her our good times with Suhel in Athens and she expressed her sorrow that Suhel was not planning to return from America to work either in Jordan or in the Medical school of Palestine. She offered us homemade "gean cherry" and cold water. We had the impression that we were visiting a traditional home in Ioannina. She invited us for dinner; we politely declined, because that evening we had to attend the official dinner for the guest speakers. "Thuk" was exited and jolly after visiting the interesting sites of the old city. The first day in Jerusalem past quickly.

Next day after my lecture, we headed for the airport to catch the flight for Larnaka airport, in Cyprus. I had scheduled to deliver a series of lectures to the members of Cyprus Medical Society. Our problem begun as soon as we reached the airport check-in point. The officer took me to his superior's office, while "Thuk" was taken in another policemen's room. The first question was why I was visiting Israel. The answer was easy: "To participate in the International Hematology meeting and deliver a lecture", I answered. My investigator continued: "If you came for a scientific meeting, why you were not attending the sessions and you were fooling around the old city?" "I wanted my son to see the beauties of your town", I answered. "Was Conzales' home an historic monument?", he ironically asked me. "No, we want to pay our respect to the mother of my colleague and friend Suhel", I replied. The police officer continued: "Did you give her any message from her son?" "Did you deliver to her any forbidden items?" "No", I answered, "just a box with chocolates. This is our custom when we visit a friend's home". The same questions were repeated again and again and the same answers were given by me. After an hour of interrogation I was obliged to undress. My clothes were scanned by a detection machine and just before the departure time of our airplane "Thuk" brought them to me.

Both exhausted and admittedly scared we departed that country with a bitter feeling. The moral of the story is to always be cautious and consider all the odds. The warm welcome and hospitality from our colleagues, in Cyprus, compensated for this unforeseen and unlucky conjecture we had to face in Israel.

5.14 Environmental Pollution or Protection?

It was midway through the 1980s. The city of Ioannina was up in arms. Concerned citizens, regardless of political party, were protesting, because the industrial company that immerses the wooden municipal electricity poles in tar to protect them from fungi and insects had set up a factory next to the riverbed into which the spring waters from the Mitsikeli mountain ran. The aquifer in those springs was the source of running water for fifty-two communities, and water is also drawn from there by two producers of bottled drinking water.

The residents were justifiably alarmed. They asked that the water be examined for traces of toxic contamination by tar. Measurements of water samples taken by the Universities of Ioannina, Munich, and Crete, as well as the General State Chemical Laboratory, revealed the presence of phenols, cresols, xyleneols, and pentachlorophenols, all cancer-causing agents found in tar. Protest marches were held, article upon article was written in the papers, experts and non-specialists took part in endless discussions on television. All with no result.

The problem began in 1968. The industrialist had been given a license to operate a wood-processing factory. Starting in 1980, however, the factory changed its operations, without a license. The owner was, you see, an influential figure. It is said that he financed many pre-election campaigns for members of Parliament, governors, and mayors. So, he had powerful protectors in all the political parties. No one bothered him, he continued producing tar for the immersion of telephone poles, and he continued polluting the environment.

One day, my secretary informed me that the industrialist in question had asked to have a meeting with me for personal reasons. I was surprised by this request for a meeting. As a doctor, however, I did not have the right to deny anyone help, no matter who it was. So, the meeting was arranged. At the appointed hour a well-dressed, short, stout man, with an aristocratic air about him, appeared at my office. He was middle-aged, and he held an expensive cigar in his hand. He introduced himself, and after giving me a short speech about my contribution to the university as a physician, teacher, and researcher, he finally came to the point as to why he was honoring me with a visit.

"I am thinking of creating an institute for environmental protection," he said, pleased with himself, and continued: "I am prepared to provide as much money as is necessary to buy the most up-to-date instruments. We have plenty of room at the factory to set up the laboratories and hire personnel for the Institute. I would like you to be the institute's first scientific director. Please let us know which departments we need to set up, the instruments necessary to run the institute, the research and assistant staff that would be required and what the yearly budget would be for it to operate smoothly. You will decide what salary you require to do this work."

I listened to him and couldn't believe what I was hearing. What colossal nerve for someone who is polluting the environment to declare that he wants to find an institute for the protection of the environment. Of course it was more than just nerve.

It was the perfect cover-up to hide his illegal activities. It reminded me of a cat who covers her feces with dirt after she defecates.

Good manners did not allow me to share these thoughts with my visitor. I reminded him that I had many teaching, departmental, and research obligations and that it would therefore not be possible for me to take on yet another responsibility.

"You will not have to spend a lot of time to direct the institute. We will hire an administrator who will take care of whatever is needed," he responded. "We only want your scientific oversight."

Of course, he did not need my scientific oversight. What he did need was my name, to be a part of his illegal actions. In spite of his insistence, I did not accept his proposal, and he left looking upset.

My refusal did not discourage the industrialist. The institute soon became a reality. Two colleagues from the University of Ioannina took on the job of directing and running it.

The protests of concerned citizens continued. In 1990, the Council of State ratified the decision of the governor of Ioannina to discontinue the operation of the immersion center. With a subsequent decision by the governor, however, the owner succeeded in getting his factory running again. There followed many license revocations, and cancellations of the revocations, as is the way of things in Greece.

The environmental pollution continued. It would take another decade before the operation of the immersion center and the institute was stopped. And why do you think this happened? The reason was the sudden death of the industrialist in a hotel, in Athens, under unspecified circumstances.

5.15 Arson Attack on Our Laboratory

The first five difficult years were over. The internal medicine department of the Ioannina University Medical School was reaching maturity. The medical wards were struggling under the weight of too many patients. It was not only people from Epirus now being treated. Our wards were hosting autoimmune rheumatic disease patients from all over the country.

An important factor in making our department operational was that it was staffed by specialists in many fields. The contribution, on both the clinical and the educational level, of physicians in the nephrology and cardiology departments was indisputable, as was the participation of volunteer specialists, such as oncologist Nikos Pavlidis and endocrinologist Giorgos Chrousos.

The immunology laboratory slowly expanded to four rooms on the ground floor of the old Hatzicostas Hospital. In the courtyard of the hospital, the laboratories of basic and pre-clinical specialization had been set up in prefab buildings. In this way, our research colleagues in the immunology laboratory could exchange scientific information with the faculty members of basic science laboratories, have the use of equipment that we lacked, and collaborate on research projects of mutual interest.

The extended space, the modernization of our equipment, and the staffing of our laboratory with technical personnel were helped along by chance occurrences. At the beginning of the decade of the 1980s, the AIDS epidemic first appeared. Our clinical service and our laboratory were designated by the Ministry of Health as "a reference center" for AIDS in northwest Greece. This enabled our laboratory to open a position for a lab technician, and to receive funding for the purchase of instruments and reagents. After a competition, we hired Cleopatra Garalea as a lab technician. She had just completed her two-year laboratory technical education. Tall, slim, and kind-hearted, she always had a smile on her face. She worked hard and did her best to continuously improve the services provided. The methods of detecting autoantibodies had all been developed at the laboratory. That gave us two advantages. First, a very low cost to carry them out, and second, extreme precision in the results obtained. At an annual European research meeting, various laboratories exchanged blood sera samples from patients, and these were examined blindly in a central European laboratory with the methods used by each laboratory to detect autoantibodies. The results obtained at our laboratory on autoantibody detection always got high grades.

The number of doctoral students working with us had increased. We chose as doctoral thesis candidates, physicians, biologists, or chemists who had excelled in their studies, had positive recommendation letters from their teachers, a good knowledge of English, and consented to work as volunteers for six months before we agreed to give them a stipend. Those who stayed with us to perform experiments and write their doctoral theses on the basis of their research understood that they would have to work long hours, become familiar with and be able to analyze current medical literature, and be cooperative with their superiors, colleagues and the lab technicians. Once they fulfilled these prerequisites, they were supported for three or four years by a small stipend or scholarship that allowed them to live independently without relying on monetary aid from their families. And where did we get this money, one might wonder. From whatever source we could find: primarily from competitive research grants from the General Secretariat of Research and Technology. The Bishop of Ioannina, Theoklitos, president of the Georgiou Stavrou Foundation, was able, through a court decision, to allocate a sum of money to support scholarships for Ph.D. candidates performing research in the laboratories of the medical school. Our studies were also funded from the research account of the Society for Epirote Studies, as in the case of Dr. Spyros Retsas, a well-known oncologist working in London who, in memory of his father, a native of Arta who fought in the mountains of Epirus during World War II, deposited a sum of money in the above research account to cover a three-year scholarship for a Ph.D. candidate working in our laboratory. In the early 1990s, we jointly applied with the departments of Biochemistry and Biology for a grant from an EEC program called "STRIDE", which was approved. With this sum of money, we were able to acquire instruments that were valuable for our research.

The research carried out at our laboratory soon brought it up to par with research labs abroad producing innovative work. Our research work attracted important scholars to us. I will mention just a few here: Aziz Charavi from Hammersmith

Hospital in London; Vladimir Vassiliev, a researcher from the Moscow Rheumatology Institute of the USSR Academy of Medicine; and Professor Rodanthi Kitridou from the University of North Carolina Medical School. In short, the immunology laboratory was teeming with young people dedicatedly working day and night and producing original research work. It was, in other words, foremost among the research laboratories in the medical school.

It was now 1986, a very difficult year. I added one more obligation to all my others. I accepted to be president of the Scientific Committee of the European Rheumatology Conference. It was scheduled to take place in June 1987, in the Peace and Friendship Stadium, in Neo Faliro, in Athens.

It was November 17, 1986, a lovely sunny morning, when I received an unexpected phone call. I was still at home, because it was a holiday. On the other end of the line was Anestis Mavridis, who was in charge of the diagnostic immunology laboratory.

"The lab has burned down," he told me, his voice trembling and out of breath.

"Burned down. How?", I asked him, alarmed.

"The immuno-chemistry room is all black," he said. "You can't see the furniture, the instruments, the chairs. They're all just one big black mass."

I didn't want to hear any more. My house was only 500 m away from the lab. In a few minutes, I was there. The picture I encountered was that of complete destruction. The laboratory was one charred mass. Fortunately, there was no one hurt. The perpetrator did his work after midnight.

We called the fire department and notified the rector's office. After examining the affected area, the fire department opined that someone had put an explosive device in the freezer.

The freezer door was at the other end of the laboratory. Both the entrance door and the freezer door had been breached. It seems that the culprit knew what he was doing. He had put the device in the place where we stored the sera of patients with autoimmune rheumatic diseases and where we kept valuable reagents.

I could not fathom what sort of sick mind had thought up this atrocity. Was it someone who wanted to hamper our research activity? Was it someone who was jealous of the progress of certain doctoral candidates? Or was it someone trying to punish us? God only knows. The instruments, the laboratory stands, and the furniture would of course be replaced. But the collection of patients' blood sera would take many years to replace.

Statements were taken and interrogations carried out. The result was one big zero. We all suspected, however, who the arsonist was. It was most probably a member of the junior faculty who, several weeks earlier, had not been promoted. But there was no clear-cut proof.

Friends of the laboratory got right to work raising funds. A good sum of money was collected. In a short time, the instruments and the furniture in our laboratory were back in place, looking as good or even better than before.

We started all over from scratch. But our enthusiasm and our desire to produce work were so great that the burning of our laboratory, instead of destroying us, made us stronger and more determined to keep producing more and better work.

5.16   Support from a Distinguished Epirote Politician

It was toward the end of 1980. The Ioannina University Medical School was taking its first small steps. Its patient care and student education were improving every day. The cooperation between clinicians and basic researchers was growing stronger. Nothing could stop its progress. There was widespread optimism and a feeling of success.

In spite of this, one great hindrance to communication between faculty members in our school was the lack of a building that would house all of its facilities. The administration was in one location, in the center of town, in one of the apartment buildings across from the office of the Prefecture of Ioannina and the Courthouse. The administrative offices of the Chairs and the lecture halls were about 500 m away from the administration building. In another part of the city, one kilometer north-east of the center, very close to the lake, in prefab buildings in the space in front of the old Hatzicostas hospital, were the basic science laboratories (anatomy, biology, biochemistry, physiology, and medical physics), and the pre-clinical course laboratories (epidemiology, hygiene, microbiology, anatomic pathology, and pharmacology). In the northern part of the city, about three kilometers away from the medical school administration building, squeezed together in the wards of the former sanatorium that became first a State Hospital and then the University Hospital, were beds for patients being treated by faculty members of internal medicine, pediatrics, orthopedic surgery, obstetrics-gynecology, and general surgery.

The distance between the buildings was a hindrance to communication, which was so important for the efficient functioning of our school. It was imperative that a suitable building be found to house the offices, the seminar rooms, the library and all the activities of our school.

After repeated meetings and consultations, a building was found: the Georgiou Stavrou Orphanage, a beautiful Greek revival building, constructed at the end of the nineteenth century on a family plot of land belonging to the donor, Georgios Stavrou, in an area called *Yiali Kafene*, very close to the old Hatzicostas Hospital. The building had a large surrounding area, fenced off by a uniquely beautiful railing. It boasted an ornate façade, a marble entranceway, and bas relief struts supporting the alcove, an arcaded inner courtyard, and many large rooms, whose walls and ceilings were adorned by elaborate paintings.

If the medical school acquired that building, most of its teaching and research activities would be accessible in a single city neighborhood. It was a unique opportunity.

The administration in charge of the National Heritage Registry under whose jurisdiction the Georgiou Stavrou building belonged, happily relinquished it to the medical school. In order to make it functional again, however, millions of drachmas needed to be spent. The university cashier's office could not cover such a large amount for expenses. There was no donor for the restoration of the building. It was urgent that one be found, but there was no one on the horizon. Sometimes in life, however, chance events can provide a solution to problems.

At that time, the Epirote politician and Minister of National Defense, Evangelos Averof, happened to be in Ioannina. I was notified by someone in his entourage that the minister was in need of my medical services. I visited him at the apartment he kept in the Tositsa Mansion. He confided to me some problems he was having with his health. He was suffering from fatigue. I did a scrupulous physical examination, I studied his lab tests and I found him in perfect health. The minister insisted, however, that we had to find the cause of his fatigue. I tried to convince him that he had to rest, to exercise, and to follow a healthy diet. He didn't listen to anything I was telling him.

He finally shared his secret with me. He showed me the injections that were invigorating him. They were a compound of vitamins B1, B6, and B12, substances that, if not medically indicated, have no therapeutic value. I explained this to him but nothing got through to him. I succumbed to his demands, and I gave him the desired injection. Its effect was immediate. He became happy as a lark. While he was still full of enthusiasm, I took the opportunity to mention to him the urgent need for the medical school to acquire the Georgiou Stavrou building. I explained to him that in order for the building to be of use to the medical school we needed to find millions of drachmas to restore it.

He did not respond to my request in words, but he acted on it at once: he immediately called the Minister of Finance and asked him to send 40 million drachmas to the office of the Prefecture of Ioannina for the restoration of the Georgiou Stavrou building. So, with a "wonder-working" injection, the medical school acquired a beautiful building to function in, worthy of its name.

5.17   The Leap to Freedom: An Albanian Colleague Defects

It was early spring, 1988. We were hosting the VIII European Workshop for Rheumatology Research at the Hilton Hotel, in Corfu. This is the most dynamic, internationally acclaimed research meeting in our field. Two hundred scientists, young and old, from all the countries in Europe, took part in the conference in order to exchange views on the latest scientific developments concerning the pathogenesis and treatment of autoimmune rheumatic diseases.

The conference was on a very tight schedule. From 8:30 in the morning to 6 in the evening the participants were confined to the hotel conference hall. The only free time was during breaks and at lunch.

The luscious greenery of the hotel garden and the calm waters of the bay stretching out before them gave the attendees a small sampling of the beauties of Corfu.

During one of the breaks, I was approached by Professor Frank Wollheim of the Lund University Medical School, in Sweden, a researcher known for his studies on understanding the pathogenesis and the development of new therapeutic interventions for scleroderma, a disease affecting the skin and other organs such as the vessels, the gastrointestinal system, the lungs, and the heart.

"In Tirana," he told me, "There is a rheumatologist at the University Hospital named Christo Mortcha. Some years ago, he worked in our section of autoimmune rheumatic diseases for a few months. He is now a docent in internal medicine and in charge of the rheumatology outpatient clinic of the University Hospital. He would very much like to work in your autoimmune rheumatic disease section for several months. He has read your studies and admires you greatly. If you accept him, you will have to support him financially."

I believed that the scientific community of our country had an obligation, most probably for its own benefit, to train scientists from neighboring countries. In this way, upon returning to their countries, they would become ambassadors for the creation of a climate of friendship, cooperation and progress in the region. Based on this thinking, I accepted that Dr. Mortcha take part in our clinical and research work.

When I returned to Ioannina from the meeting in Corfu, I was able to secure room and board for our visitor with the help of the Metropolitan of Ioannina, who gave him a room with a bathroom at the Ioannina nursing home. With money from the special account at the Society for Epirote Studies, we provided our visitor with a small monthly stipend for his expenses.

In the spring of 1989, Dr. Christo Mortcha appeared at my office in the Hatzicostas Hospital, with no prior notice. He was a tall, upright, well-dressed gentleman who spoke perfect English. He looked like a European doctor.

He quickly adapted to the routines of the Autoimmune Rheumatic Diseases Section. He was polite, discreet, and pleasant and became friends with the physicians and colleagues in the department. His adjustment to our country was perfect.

One day, about two months after his arrival, he very politely asked me if I could invite his family to Ioannina for a weekend.

"I want them to see how free people live, the advances in your country and the natural beauty here," he said to me.

I found his request reasonable. The invitation was sent. The response was immediate. His wife and two daughters arrived for a visit. They too spoke perfect English.

"Did you go to an English school in Tirana?", I asked them.

They told me that Christo's father had studied for many years in America, and that he was their teacher.

On the weekend, we showed them the cultural and natural treasures of the city and gave them the opportunity to taste local dishes. They all seemed happy.

The surprise came on Monday morning. The family had gathered outside the door of my house.

"Why haven't you left yet?", I asked.

"We have decided to stay in Greece," they answered. "We're not going back. Do whatever you like with us."

The truth is I was shocked. I was at a loss for words. I didn't expect this development. Whereas I had planned to send a trained colleague back to a neighboring country to offer his services there, I suddenly had his whole family under my charge. This was something that had never happened to me before. I soon decided I had to take action, first in order to legalize them, that is, to begin the procedure for granting political asylum, and then to find them lodgings. As soon as we submitted the necessary applications for political asylum, the Mortcha family was held in custody for several days by the police. I got in touch with all the government agencies in the city—the governor, the mayor, the Metropolitan—and the family was released. They were granted political asylum.

The Metropolitan, always ready to help, gave them an apartment to stay in for free. Christo's wife found a job. His children, the same age as mine, were enrolled in the same Greek school. The progress of the entire family was impressive. Nothing got in their way. They were overjoyed and energized by the freedom of speech, thought, and action in Greece. In record time they all learned Greek. Christo took exams and got his Albanian Medical Diploma recognized. At first he was appointed to serve as a physician in a rural district. He took more exams and was recognized as a rheumatology specialist in Greece. The family was moving further and further up in the world every day.

Today, they live in Athens. They are financially comfortable and, most important of all, very happy. Every time I see them they never fail to express their gratitude for the help I gave them during that difficult time in their life. I am touched by the genuine expression of their feelings.

5.18   Educator Abroad

5.18.1   Sabbatical Year in France

One day in the late 1980s, I got a call from Professor Pierre Youinnou informing me that the National French Committee for the Selection of Visiting Professors had selected me as *professeur associé* to serve for one year in the immunology laboratory of the Brest University Medical School. They wanted me to organize their studies on Sjögren's syndrome. I thanked him for the honor, and I told him that I would gladly take on the responsibility if I could spend only 10 days out of every month in Brest. My department was still too young and my physical presence there, I felt, was useful. My terms were accepted, and I soon began my tenure in Brest.

During my first ten days in Brest, I was a guest at the Youinnous' home, a three-story house with a relatively big yard, in which trees, plants, and grass were growing with no particular care from the owners. I had the whole attic to myself. There was a double sofa bed there, a small table and a chair, and there were beautiful paintings hanging on every inch of the walls, as there were on the walls in the rest of the house. Véronique, Pierre's wife, was a superb abstract painter. She painted for her own satisfaction; she never exhibited or sold her work. She has gifted us many pieces of her artwork.

In the sitting room the walls were covered by bookcases, filled with books of literature (Photo 5.7). Another piece of furniture contained vinyl records. A record

Photo 5.7 Author and
Professor Pierre Youinnou at
the latter's house

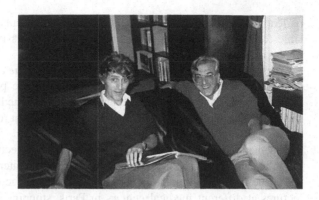

player on top of a buffet was constantly playing opera music. Pierre was a Maria
Callas lover. TV was not allowed at the Youinnou house.

Their hospitality was incomparable. Their food was delicious and it was served on
a strict schedule, always at 1 p.m. and at 7 p.m. All the family members—4 children
(two boys and two girls) and the parents had fixed seats at the table; the visitor was
seated next to the pater familias. During my stay at their house, Pierre would drive
me back and forth to the laboratory in his car. He drove like a maniac. I have to admit
I was scared. On all my subsequent trips to Brest I stayed at the *Hôtel de la Paix,* a
hotel located within walking distance from the Brest University Medical Center.

My first days in Brest were for orientation. In the lab I met all the personnel,
including secretaries, technicians, and the other staff members. Every member of
the lab outlined his or her research work. Afterward, appointments were scheduled
to meet the professors of internal medicine, nephrology, pulmonology, and rheumatology, all of whom were interested in learning about autoimmune rheumatic diseases.
They too explained to me their research interests. Together, by year's end, we had
three clinical laboratory papers ready for publication.

At the end of the meetings with the professors, a young pathologist, a Ph.D.
student, was introduced to me. I was assigned to plan and supervise his research work
toward his Ph.D. He was an introverted, unassuming sort. Throughout our conversation, I evaluated the extent of his knowledge on Sjögren's syndrome. I recommended
to him a list of research papers he should study before we planned his experimental
work. In the next few months, we completed a study on corneal epithelial cells from
patients with Sjögren's syndrome and normal individuals. This study revealed that
the corneal epithelial cells of patients with Sjögren's syndrome had an activated
phenotype. Nuclear and cellular autoantigens as well as other immune-regulating
proteins were inappropriately expressed on the surface of these cells. Our findings,
in combination with previous histopathologic findings revealing that the inflammatory cells are localized around the epithelia of organs affected by the syndrome, as
well as the findings of immunopathology studies demonstrating that immunoregula-
tory molecules are inappropriately expressed on the surface of epithelial cells of the

patients' salivary glands, indicated that these cell populations appear to be responsible for the initiation and perpetuation of autoaggressive lesions observed in the organs affected by Sjögren's syndrome.

These findings led me to coin the name *autoimmune epithelitis* for the Sjögren's syndrome entity, a name which is descriptive of the pathobiologic processes of this entity. In addition, these initial findings stimulated us to plan and execute a series of experiments that further proved the significant role of epithelial cells in the pathogenesis of the syndrome.

Another pleasant responsibility in Brest was the lectures I delivered, based on our clinical and laboratory research. The amphitheater was packed with young colleagues, and you could see the thirst for knowledge on their faces. I also gave lectures at different medical centers in Paris, stopping over for a day during my flights from Greece to Brest. In Paris, I stayed at the house of Pierre's sister.

The sabbatical year also gave me time for pleasure and relaxation. I enjoyed the French cuisine and in particular delicacies such as soupe à l'oignon, steak tartare, bouillabaisse, bœuf bourguignon, and fruits de mer. In my free time, Pierre and I visited different areas of Brittany. I remember in particular a visit to his mother, who lived in an old mansion in the center of the city of Duoarnenez, where Pierre was born and raised. Pierre's father was the local physician. His mother, despite her advanced age, was decorously dressed, polite and had a strong sense of hospitality. The Youinnous and I also attended opera performances, in Rennes. The fear and the adrenaline released in me because of Pierre's driving managed to wipe out the euphoria created by the music. I tried once or twice to swim in the Atlantic Ocean, but my Mediterranean nature wouldn't permit me to wade even a few meters into those unwelcoming waters. Overall, however, I fully enjoyed my time in Brest.

5.18.2 Australian Days

It was May 1991. I was flying to Sydney, Australia. I had been honored with the European-Australian Award for my contribution to the understanding of the pathogenesis of autoimmune rheumatic diseases. Professor Nik Christophidis had nominated me for this honor. I didn't know that colleague, but searching his curriculum and bibliography, I found out that he was a gerontologist, studying methotrexate metabolism in the elderlies. During my visit in Australia, I was assigned the task of teaching in university hospitals and biomedical Institutions.

In the flight to Australia only two people were in business class, me and a tall, middle-aged man. I had not bought my ticket myself. It was part of the honorary invitation. My income, moreover, did not allow such luxuries.

My fellow traveler was wandering around the aisles of the airplane; he didn't stay in one place for a second. He seemed to want to talk. The trip was long, with no end in sight. Twenty-two hours. We soon began talking. The minute he opened his mouth I understood that he was from the north of Greece.

"Where you headed, young man?".

"To Sydney," I answered.

"You got people there?", he asked me.

I told him who I was and explained the purpose of my trip to him. The more we talked, the more curious I became about who he was. He was more than glad to share his life story with me.

He was an orphan, and grew up working for some relatives for a few scraps of food and a straw mattress to sleep on. In the early 1950s, when he was thirteen, he and some other villagers went to try their luck working in Australia.

"We traveled in a rotten old ship. I stayed on deck the whole trip. I'd paid next to nothing for my ticket. Soon as we got to Australia, they put me on a train. God only knew where we were heading. My first job was herding lambs to be slaughtered. I didn't like that job. As soon as I learned a few words of English I picked myself up and went to Sydney. I did every kind of work you can imagine. At first, I lived in a basement room. The landlady was Chinese. She made spring rolls and sold them to Chinese restaurants. In the afternoon when I was off work, I tried to help her. I wanted to learn her trade. I married the daughter of one of my fellow villagers. We started making spring rolls together. Soon people heard about us. At the end of it all, our work from the house turned into a big industry. Today, we're the largest manufacturers of frozen foods in Australia: two factories here and one in Romania. My son-in-law directs the one in Romania. He studied engineering there. He's from our village. He married my daughter."

I won't continue telling you about my dialog with my cabin mate or about all his property in Greece, but I do want to share with you, dear reader, his life experience, which is not at all unique. I have encountered it many times with Greek immigrants to Australia. The lesson is that for someone to get ahead, he needs to first be helped along by his natural intelligence, and to not mind hard work. He needs to keep at it, to be reliable, to be cooperative and to take advantage, in the good sense of the term, of opportunities. With those qualities, my co-passenger succeeded in becoming one of the richest Greeks in Australia. He owns a television station and is the president of the biggest football team in Australia.

That is one side of the coin from my experience with Greek people in Australia.

I taught in all the university hospitals and institutes of Sidney, Melbourne, and Adelaide. In Sydney, my good friend and colleague Professor Steve Krilis, internationally known researcher on the anti-phospolipid syndrome, hosted me at his home. He and his wife, Philippa, treated me as if I were a member of their family. They took me to exceptionally good fish restaurants and performances and gave a dinner at their home to which prominent Greek-Australians were invited. At that dinner, I had the unique opportunity to meet Archbishop Stylianos, a highly progressive priest and talented poet. In Melbourne, I met Professor Nick Cristophidis a dedicated pharmacologist and his wife, a sculptor. Nick did me the honor of attending almost all my lectures in Melbourne.

In addition to scientific lectures, I was invited by various patient associations to discuss with them different aspects of autoimmune rheumatic diseases.

One of these meetings has remained indelibly etched in my mind. There, I saw the other side of the coin in Australia.

The lecture room was packed. Many listened standing up. When my talk was over, a group of people approached me. They told me they were from Ioannina, and that they represented an Epirote association, and they invited me to their club. As we were leaving the lecture hall, another group from Ioannina came up to me and also invited me for a meal. I explained to them that I had already accepted an invitation by a group from Ioannina. I thought it was the same group. But things were not as I believed.

The club we went to was in a semi-basement space about fifty square meters in size. The smoky smell of roasted meat hit us immediately. The grill was in the corner of the room. The tables were arranged in the shape of the Greek letter Pi (Π). The tablecloths, yellow with black stripes, reminded me of Greek village taverns in the decade of the 1950s. They put me at the head of the table. They started serving wine from a large keg. A middle-aged man with classic Epirote features, the president of the club, I believe, stood up to make a toast and welcome me. But instead of the usual polite statements, it was clear from his very first words that he was very hostile to the medical establishment in Greece. It seems my presence awoke unpleasant memories in him. He let loose a torrent of insulting words such as "dishonest," "ignorant," "crass," and I don't remember what else. The gentleman had forgotten that his adopted country was honoring me for my scientific contributions. I couldn't contain myself. I stood up and interrupted him.

"I know and continue to believe that one of the main characteristics of the Epirotes is their hospitality. But, sadly, I now see that when they find themselves in a foreign country this attribute disappears. I thank you for the invitation, but I cannot share a meal with slanderers. I bid you good day and wish you all the best."

My reaction shocked them. They ran after me, begging me to stay. When I was back in my room, having now calmed down, I began to make excuses for them. Those people felt like rejected children. Their country drove them away, uprooted them. Why should they feel happy when confronted with a successful compatriot? So they turned against everyone, right or wrong.

The following day, I spoke with a colleague of mine of Greek origin and tried to understand what sort of Epirotes were represented by that club. He explained that there were two Epirote organizations and, smiling, he then said:

"From what you told me, I'm pretty sure that the club that invited you was the one we call 'Little Moscow.'"

5.19 Acquiring New Equipment: The Perils of Overzealousness

It was the beginning of the decade of the 1990s. The internal medicine wards had moved from the third-world conditions of the Hatzicostas Hospital to the comfortable luxury of the newly built University Hospital in Dourouti, an area five kilometers outside the city limits of Ioannina. The patients of the internal medicine wards were housed in two wings on the third floor, and the patients of the pulmonology section in one wing on the second floor. All three wings were located in the first of three hospital towers, while on the first floor of the third tower the cardiology section and the ICU for coronary diseases were set up. The patients were put up in single, double, and four-bed rooms.

On the main floor of the hospital there was a large lecture hall and an amphitheater that held 250 people, with the latest optical and acoustic equipment. All the laboratories were well equipped, but the radiology laboratory was missing a CT scanner. It had been installed at the Hatzicostas Hospital to be used by the departments operating there. But there's nothing more permanent than something temporary, as they say. So while the medical school wards moved to Dourouti Hospital, the CT scanner remained in the old hospital.

One day, I don't remember exactly when a colleague telephoned me from the Ygeia Hospital in Athens. Medical ethics do not permit me to reveal the names of the physician or the patient. Suffice it to say, however, that the patient was a well-known businessman with interests abroad.

The doctors treating him had suspected, based on his symptoms and his clinical and laboratory tests, that he was suffering from an inflammation of his blood vessels called vasculitis. My colleague did not hide from me the fact that he was calling me on the advice of physicians at the Mayo Clinic, whom they had previously contacted to help with the diagnosis and treatment of his patient. Two or three days later the patient was moved to our department. A thorough examination uncovered the culprit. It was an ancient kind of belt that he wore day and night to keep his innards in place to prevent strangulation of his inguinal hernia. But the pressure from the belt he was wearing hindered the flow of blood from his lower limbs to his heart. The inadequate blood flow caused the formation of clots in the veins of the patient's lower limbs, and those clots came loose from time to time and became attached to blood vessels of the lung. That is to say, the patient was suffering from relapsing pulmonary embolisms. These caused fever, coughing, blood in the sputum and gave a false picture of vasculitis. The belt was removed, the patient was treated with anticoagulants, and in a matter of days our visitor was ready to leave. Before he left the hospital, he came to my office to express his gratitude to me, and like the excellent businessman that he was, he calculated what the bill would have been in a loud voice:

"If I had gone to a hospital in America, I would have spent thousands and thousands of dollars," he said. "I saved that money, so I would like to make it available to you for the purchase of equipment to improve the operation of your hospital."

Needless to say, I was very pleased with his proposal. I immediately thought of the hospital's need for a CT scanner. I explained to him the value of that instrument for arriving at a diagnosis and monitoring the response to therapy of various illnesses, and before I had even finished my proposal, he accepted most happily to buy the CT scanner.

The patient went soon afterward to visit the president of the hospital board to announce to him his intention to make this donation. And what do you think the gentleman in charge of the operation of our University Hospital said? Sit down and hold onto your seats.

"There's no need for you to make a donation. The government will buy the CT scanner."

And he foolishly explained: "If, on behalf of the hospital, I accept your donation, it will make Professor Moutsopoulos even more powerful." That fool, jealous of my performance as physician, teacher, and researcher, deprived the hospital of the opportunity to acquire a very valuable instrument.

I don't think I need to comment further on the malicious and thoughtless behavior of the president of our hospital. Unfortunately, many of those governing our institutions have a similar mentality. They occupy positions of responsibility not because they are educated and competent but because they make promises to everyone about everything, and in this way, they promote favor-swapping and corruption in government-run facilities.

The businessman, upset and confused by the malice of the leader of our hospital, came to see me again. He recounted their discussion to me. He was dumbfounded. But he did not let this discourage him from making a donation. He asked me to suggest another piece of equipment that would be used solely for the department I was in charge of. I was ready with a proposal. I recommended that he buy us an angiography instrument for carrying out angiograms on coronary arteries.

The proposal was implemented immediately. And that's how angiograms began to be performed in Ioannina. The flow of patients from Ioannina to Athens to undergo this life-saving examination soon came to an end once and for all.

5.20 The Beginning of the End of the Ioannina Era

More than ten years had passed since I took up the Chair of Internal Medicine at the Ioannina University Medical School. Our department was steadily growing. New faculty members and consultants in internal medicine and section heads were elected and appointed. From a one-man show, our department developed into a fully staffed contemporary, diagnostic, therapeutic, educational, and research environment, not only in internal medicine but also in the majority of internal medicine specialties. All new faculty members had been trained abroad. In addition to autoimmune rheumatic disease, pulmonology, and hematology experts, new faculty members were elected and appointed in internal medicine, nephrology, gastroenterology, endocrinology, oncology, and cardiology.

Some members of our department went on to find jobs in other medical facilities. One rheumatologist became an assistant professor at the department of Medicine of Patras University; another was appointed consultant rheumatologist at Papanikolaou Hospital in Thessaloniki, and an excellent clinician became the director of the Governmental department of Internal Medicine at Hatzicostas Hospital. Four others, after some years of training abroad, also advanced their careers. One became director of the endocrinology section of the Athens Polyclinic; another was appointed a faculty member of the ICU at Evangelismos Hospital, in Athens; still another, a productive pulmonologist, was moved from our staff to the pulmonary section at Evangelismos

Hospital, while the fourth was elected associate professor in internal medicine at the department of Thessaly Medical School, in Larissa. In other words, our department became a supplier of scientists to other medical institutions.

Patients from all over Greece and Cyprus with symptoms and signs of autoimmune rheumatic diseases were seeking appointments at our outpatient clinic for diagnosis and therapy. Our research contributions to the field of autoimmune rheumatic diseases, with an emphasis on the clinical spectrum and pathogenetic mechanisms of Sjögren's syndrome, were increasingly recognized and acknowledged by the international scientific community.

The production of new knowledge from the research laboratory was receiving considerable recognition in Greece and abroad. At the Greek medical conferences, our young researchers frequently won the Papastamatis Award, a distinction given for innovative research. The same scenario played out in annual research meetings held in European countries.

In 1987, the European Rheumatology Conference honored me with the Alessandro Robecci Award for my contribution to understanding the pathogenesis of autoimmune diseases. Various universities in Europe and America also invited me as a visiting professor. European and American conferences honored me as a plenary speaker. Our department, because of its good scientific reputation, was given the task of organizing two international meetings, in 1988 and 1991. The first was the European Workshop for Research I mentioned earlier and was held at the Hilton Hotel in Corfu, and the second, on Sjögren's syndrome, was held at the building of the Society for Epirote Studies, in Ioannina (Photo 5.8).

Photo 5.8 A scientific session of the III International Symposium on Sjögren's Syndrome held in Ioannina, Greece

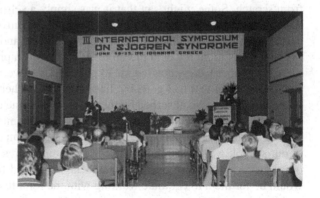

5.21   Candidate for Professorship at the Athens University Medical School

I believed the time had come to declare my candidacy for professor at the Athens University Medical School. Toward the end of the 1980s, the position of professor of medicine at the Athens University Medical School, previously held by Professor Giorgos Daïkos, was announced. I decided to apply for that position. I thought that I would be elected to this post since all the faculty members of the department of Internal Medicine there were familiar with my clinical, scientific, and administrative qualifications. Furthermore, starting in the early 1980s, Professor Daïkos and his department had developed a joint educational program with me and my department for our students and residents. Twice a year, we held a clinical pathology conference somewhere in Greece. At those meetings, interesting medical cases were used to teach differential diagnosis, diagnosis, and treatment of a certain group of diseases, using as a paradigm a patient's clinical and pathological history. In one meeting a resident from our department would present an interesting medical case, and a specialist from Professor Daïkos' department would discuss it. At the next meeting, we would do the reverse. In that way, the students of both medical schools came into contact with many different teachers of medicine. My interest in applying for the job was further aroused because certain professors at the Athens University Medical School, who were well-known for their clinical and scientific contributions to our field, urged me to apply.

The reader may wonder, seeing as I had succeeded in creating such a well-functioning department in Ioannina, why I would want to move to the Athens University Medical School and again organize clinical and research laboratories from scratch. Some might say that it was simply a self-serving move, because the Athens University Medical School was the foremost university in the country. But it was also the school that taught me the art of medicine and the love of my profession. My highest aspiration would therefore be to become a professor at that school. But there were other factors that led me to pursue this move.

In the decade that had gone by, the young researchers who had come of age in Ioannina could not be absorbed by the internal medicine department of the Ioannina University Medical School. There were already many members of the junior faculty serving there. The internal medicine department, in comparison to other departments in our school, was already overstaffed. The younger researchers were not ready to organize departments in other medical schools around the country. The best thing would be for them to continue working with me for a few more years before taking up a higher academic position, even though this meant moving to another university.

Another factor that made me want to become professor at the Athens University Medical School was the insufficient funding we had in Ioannina, compared to the Athens University Medical School. The truth is that in our country whoever is closest to centers of power enjoys the most benefits.

One more reason that pushed me to create another department was that I believed that I had now given as much as I could to the Ioannina University Medical School. It was time for someone younger in age, but also a mature and well-trained colleague, to take over the position of professor and chairman.

In the end, I applied for the professorship in Athens. The other candidate for the Chair was the interim director of the department, a colleague more than ten years older than me, but without significant scientific accomplishments.

When I remember what I went through, at that time, as a candidate for a professorship in Athens, it still upsets me. My experience in Athens was in no way comparable to the way I was treated as a candidate for professor of internal medicine at the Ioannina University Medical School. Most of the electors in the Ioannina University Medical School were individuals who had spent many years teaching at universities abroad. By contrast, the majority of electors in Athens did everything they could to discourage and deter every qualified candidate who was not already serving in their school. In order to improve the international profile of a university school, however, those in charge of electing new faculty members need to offer financial and scientific incentives to attract the best candidates, not to discourage them from being candidates. Despite the fact that my candidacy had been supported by the internationally known professors of the Athens University Medical School, the other candidate was elected.

This was the first significant failure in my academic life. I could not come to terms with the fact that I had lost the election to a candidate whose academic credentials were far inferior to mine. This unjustified failure was extremely distressing to me, and a month or two later I began to suffer from insomnia, tachycardia, weight loss, and other disturbances, heralding the onset of an overactive thyroid gland. This was the second attack on my body by an autoimmune disease. The first was when I had Guillain-Barré syndrome in late adolescence. My siblings also suffered from these autoimmune syndromes, so it was now fairly obvious that the distress caused by my academic failure, combined with my genetic predisposition for autoimmune diseases, led to the activation of my immune system in an attack on my thyroid gland. Thanks to the meticulous care of Dr. Dionysius Ikkos, the best endocrinologist in our country at that time, the disease was treated.

Fortunately for me, none of this distracted me from my goals, the optimal care of my patients, the education of younger colleagues, and the production of new scientific knowledge. I simply dug in further and began new collaborations. One of these was with Professor Sakarellos, an organic chemist and his scientific team at our university. Together we studied and tried to uncover the exact position on autoantigens where autoantibodies (antibodies directed against autoantigens) would bind. This area of the autoantigen is called an epitope and usually consists of 6–8 amino acids. There were three goals to these studies: (a) to use these epitopes to develop cheap, sensitive, and specific diagnostic tests for the detection of autoantibodies in the sera of patients with autoimmune diseases; (b) to study the structure of the epitopes and use this to identify the exogenous agent that triggers the immune system to react against its own antigens and initiate autoimmune disease; and (c) to ameliorate autoimmune reactivity by administering these epitopes intra-nasally, bound to a carrier molecule, to patients with autoimmune diseases with the specific autoantibody.

Several years had now passed since the time I failed to be elected professor at Athens University Medical School, when I got a call from Professor Charis Roussos, the chairman of the ICU at Evangelismos Hospital, in Athens. He had returned to Greece from Canada only two or three years earlier and had been one of my strongest supporters during my previous candidacy for the professorship in the Athens University Medical School. He informed me that the position of professor of pathophysiology was declared open and urged me to apply. He tried his best to convince me that this position was more suitable for my work since this department, in addition to its clinical service, had a large laboratory space where I could continue my immunology experiments. He also informed me that a large proportion of the electors were positively disposed to my getting the position. I thanked him for his concern, and I asked him to allow me some time to seriously think over whether I wanted to again go through a demeaning and traumatic experience. Charis' telephone call was followed by telephone calls from other senior professors at the Athens University Medical School. All of them encouraged me to apply. As it was now close to the cut-off date, I decided to declare my candidacy. This time things were much easier. I received twenty-nine out of thirty votes from the electoral body. And a new era in my academic life was about to begin.

Chapter 6
Department of Pathophysiology, Athens University Medical School

6.1 Assuming the Professorship

In November of 1993, I took up my new position. The dean of the medical school introduced me to my colleagues in the department of Pathophysiology. Then it was my turn to speak to them. I summarized for them the way I wanted our clinical section and research laboratory to function. I reminded them all that my main goal was excellent and up-to-date teaching of the students and the physicians in specialty training, through first-rate hospital care for patients, plus the production of new knowledge. During that first meeting, we were all restrained and somewhat frightened, I would say; me, because I was feeling anxious about whether I would be able to create a more contemporary department of Pathophysiology with a research laboratory turning out innovative work, and my colleagues because they did not know what to expect from their new director.

After that brief meeting, they arranged for me to visit the laboratory and the patient wards. The previous director, Menis Fertakis, who had lost his professorship to me, showed me around with great tact, sincerity, and respect. The laboratory had been founded by Professor Vasilis Angelopoulos, a hematologist, twenty years earlier. My visit there made clear to me that Professor Angelopoulos had unique administrative abilities and the vision for a contemporary university department. There were laboratories for all the sections of internal medicine. Our laboratory was like new, but the instruments were out-of-date. I made a note of which laboratories I would select to house the colleagues, who had come with me from Ioannina.

I did not come alone. I was followed by three generations of researchers, who had developed scientifically in the department of Internal Medicine and the immunology laboratory of the Ioannina University Medical School.

Professor Fotini Skopouli, who by that time had become my life companion, decided to give up her position as associate professor of Internal Medicine at the Ioannina University Medical School and follow me to Athens. Because of our close relationship, however, we decided not to work in the same place. We tried, through our example, to ensure that there would be no conflict of interest, a choice that is

H. M. Moutsopoulos, *Passion for Excellence*, Springer Biographies,
https://doi.org/10.1007/978-3-031-14128-7_6

rarely made in our country. At first, Fotini, on a leave of absence, helped to set up the immunology laboratory of the department of Pathophysiology. When her leave expired, she was appointed director of the internal medicine department at the Evgenidio University Hospital. Not long afterward, she was elected professor of internal medicine and immunology in the department of Nutrition and Dietetics Studies of Harokopio University.

Athanasios Tzioufas, Panayotis Vlachoyiannopoulos, and Menelaos Manoussakis, who had been trained in Ioannina as internists, or rheumatologists and had produced high-quality clinical and research work, also followed me to Athens. They were my second generation of scientists.

I assumed the chairmanship of a department and a laboratory with a large number of personnel in every specialty, with lab technicians, and two secretaries. They had been used to working a certain way for many years. I had to figure out how I could get us to work together in the way that I preferred. I was sure I could make our department an excellent, up-to-date clinical center with high-standard teaching for students and young physicians, and at the same time a renowned research environment for the production of new knowledge. This was, in other words, a different kind of challenge for me than I had at the University of Ioannina. There, we could say that an uncultivated patch of land became, with my help, a productive field. Here in Athens, the land had been cultivated, but in a different way, for many years.

From the very first moment, I understood that the secretaries, Pola Papadopoulou and Voula Korba (Photo 6.1), were ready to help with the task I was undertaking. This was not expressed in actual words but became unambiguously clear in the way actions have of speaking. During my entire tenure in Athens, they were the pillars of our department. Pola retired in 2002 and Voula continues to ungrudgingly put up with the idiosyncrasies of her boss.

Photo 6.1 Department secretaries Voula Korba and Pola Papadopoulou

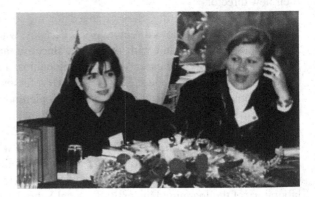

6.2 First Visit to the Athens University Laïko General Hospital

The patient wards of the department of Pathophysiology were located on the fourth floor of the hospital. The department's laboratories were on the third floor of the basic science building and communicated directly with the patient wards.

Before I went to the patient ward of our department, I thought it would be a good idea to have a thorough look at the rest of the hospital. I had been a resident at one of the university departments in that hospital before I left for specialization in America. From the first glance I could tell that the hospital had not been modernized in the twenty years that had passed. The patients were crammed into rooms with a large number of beds, which forced them to be so close together that it was almost unsanitary. Very few rooms had washrooms or bathrooms for the patients. The male patients were reminded of conditions during their military service, with many soldiers sharing washrooms and bathrooms. The most disappointing part of it all, however, was the Paleolithic infrastructure of the diagnostic laboratories. When I asked my colleagues: "Where do you perform modern diagnostic tests?". They answered: "We send them to private laboratories." "How do you choose those diagnostic centers?", I asked. "An administrative officer keeps a list by order of which centers have priority," they replied.

In this country, where everyone is suspicious of everyone else, it is not possible for a physician serving in a state hospital to choose a laboratory. If he/she systematically sends patients to the same laboratory, very few people will believe that he/she has chosen the best one, since no objective evaluation is possible. Most people will be sure that the physician is on the take.

I will not hide from you the fact that this first visit was disheartening. I began wondering if I had done the right thing by abandoning the impeccable guest lodgings and technical infrastructure of the Ioannina University Hospital, and if I would again end up in conditions similar to those under which I had to work in the Hatzicostas Hospital. But my tenacious nature emboldened me to start over again from scratch. I have to confess, however, dear reader, that it took me many years until I stopped feeling depressed every time I walked through the corridors of the Laïko General Hospital on my way to visit patients on the fourth floor.

Many things have changed in the intervening years, but many changes have yet to be made. The infrastructure of the hospital was modernized, but important instruments are still lacking, such as magnetic resonance imaging and positron emission tomography machines. I don't believe they will be acquired in the near future.

A wing was created with accommodations where a few lucky patients could enjoy treatment under tolerable conditions. Doctors would compete to get their patients a place there. To avoid misunderstandings, those beds were handled by the chief administrator of the hospital. This served many purposes.

The number of beds in the ICU increased and their infrastructure improved, but still the number was low in comparison to the overall number of patient beds in the hospital.

New departments were developed, not based on the needs of the hospital, but on the needs of those who had easy access to the Ministry of Health. But important departments were not instituted and developed, such as thoracic and cardiac surgery, neurosurgery, neurology, and psychiatry, essential specialties for the harmonious functioning of a university hospital.

6.3   Separating the Wheat from the Chaff

I set up in-person meetings with all the senior and junior faculty members in our clinical service and our laboratory. I wanted to learn from each of them what their teaching, clinical, and research interests were. For this reason, I got their permission to record our discussions. The meetings were going along smoothly. I began to get a picture of the colleagues I would be working with.

Then all of a sudden, a surprise came. It was the turn of the last faculty member I had to see.

He came into my office with what I would call an easy, almost impolite, air. In so many words, he announced to me that he was not doing any work at the clinical service, nor was he teaching or doing night shifts, but was serving as the director of the internal medicine department of a large private hospital. When I heard his statement, I couldn't believe my ears. I repeated it to make sure I had heard correctly. In any event, I had recorded it.

"Are you an unpaid worker?", I asked him.

"No, I draw a proper salary," he answered, "if you could call a puny few thousand drachmas a salary," he added.

I was truly dumbfounded. I had nothing else to say. I sent him on his way, but I knew immediately what I had to do. I sent an urgent memorandum to the administrative authorities of the medical school and the university outlining what had happened in careful detail.

Several days later, I received a telephone call from one of the senior professors.

"What have you done to our colleague?", he said.

"I didn't do anything," I answered. "I think he did something to himself. It was my duty to report the resulting violation to the administrative authorities, so that the responsibility would no longer rest with me," I said, and continued: "If the administration does not act within a reasonable amount of time, then I will send my report to the district attorney."

My interlocutor tried in every way he could to persuade me to cancel my memorandum. It seems that some old-school professors believe they can impose their viewpoint on anyone, even if it is not legal. He did not succeed in convincing me to recant.

The colleague in question heard the news from his protector and understood that I was not just playing. So he found a solution. He resigned from his position as assistant professor of pathophysiology.

The first battle was won. I believe this was a useful lesson for everyone serving in the pathophysiology department.

Two more members of our department followed his example and resigned. Both held positions at other hospitals, one as director of internal medicine and the other as director of the immunology laboratory.

We very quickly organized and began implementing the post-graduate educational program. We used the same program as in Ioannina. Everyone, teachers and students, took part. They did not simply attend, they participated actively.

There was, however, one particular colleague who was always absent from those classes. After noting down her repeated absences, I decided to send her a note asking her to explain why she was not participating in the post-graduate courses. In the note I also asked if her absence was indicative of her disapproval of the level or the contents of the courses, and I ended by saying that her comments would be most helpful in improving our post-graduate program and making it attractive to everyone.

I received an unexpected answer. In a formal note she informed me that she could not attend our classes because there was a conflict with her private office hours, which were at the same time.

I was shocked by her nerve. But I made no decisions and left the matter at that.

Two months later, I don't remember exactly when that same colleague sent me another formal note whose style and content were unacceptable. She accused a post-graduate student, who was studying the blood of patients with AIDS, of carelessly spilling a patient's blood serum on her laboratory workbench, and she concluded by saying that if she developed AIDS, I would be morally and legally responsible.

I called her to my office. I asked her if she had written that note herself.

"Of course," she answered.

My next question was if she knew how long the AIDS virus could live on a laboratory workbench surface. Her answer was not clear. Next, I informed her that the serum used by that doctoral candidate had been de-activated with heat treatment, that is, the virus had been killed and was therefore harmless. So, it was not possible that the blood serum could cause AIDS.

"Unfortunately, my dear colleague," I continued, "your letter makes indisputably clear three things: first, that you are against research on AIDS. I will inform the Movement for the Freedom of Greek Homosexuals of your position, and I leave you to work things out directly with them. Second, in spite of the fact that you are a micro-biologist, you are unaware of how the AIDS virus is transmitted, something which any educated person in our country knows. I will inform the Society of Greek Micro-biologists about your insufficient training. And third, the rude and provocative tone of your letter is unacceptable to me. I will pass it on to the academic administration of our school and recommend that you receive exemplary punishment."

My comments caused her to turn ten shades paler. She was clearly scared. Not long after our meeting I found her resignation on my desk.

6.4   Reorganization of the Department of Pathophysiology

When I took over the administration, the department of Pathophysiology had eight sections. Its organization dated back to the time Professor Vasilis Angelopoulos was the director. The strongest section was hematology, staffed by an associate professor, two assistant professors, two physicians doing hematology training, and a technician. The second most active section was gastroenterology, staffed by an associate professor, an assistant professor, a lecturer, and one physician in gastroenterology training. The third section was endocrinology, staffed by an assistant professor, two physicians in endocrinology training, and a technician. The fourth section was for rheumatic disease, headed by an associate professor and two trainees. The other sections, such as nephrology, pulmonology, infectious diseases, and metabolic diseases had only one faculty member without trainees. Twelve young physicians were in training in internal medicine. The majority of the medical sections had an outpatient clinic. The laboratory faculty members were two clinical pathologists, two biochemists, two nuclear physicists, and three laboratory technicians.

The inpatient clinical service was run in an outdated manner. Each faculty member was in charge of a hospital ward hosting six to eight patients. This organization was primarily for the benefit of the head physician of the ward but was not useful for optimal patient care, or for training young physicians and medical students. This arrangement had to change right away. I called a meeting with all the clinical faculty members of the department and I explained to them the new way the clinical service would be organized and run from then on. Three teams would be developed: the red, the blue, and the green. Each team would be headed by a faculty member, two physicians in training, and four medical students. The heads of the teams would serve for two or three months, according to the availability of faculty members, and then another faculty member would take over the responsibility of the team. I would do the chief of service rounds on Monday, Wednesday, and Friday from 10.30 a.m. till noon. The objective of the chief of service rounds was three-fold: (a) to see that the clinical service was running smoothly, (b) to assist in the diagnosis of difficult cases, and (c) for the physicians of the team to become familiar with his medical thinking and take advantage of his knowledge. Some of the senior faculty members whispered: "What are we going to do when we are not in clinical service"? I answered: "(a) you will do research; (b) you will update your teaching material, and (c) you will improve the functioning of the outpatient clinic you are responsible for running." Before concluding our meeting, I made clear that the administration of the department strongly condemns and will not tolerate under the table payments by patients to faculty members or to any physicians in our clinical service. Furthermore, I stated that the only way a faculty member would be promoted was through exemplary care of patients, dedication to teaching students and trainees, and the production of new knowledge through clinical and/or laboratory research.

Next, I had to modernize and update the operation of the laboratory. Unfortunately, since the research was not being performed, many laboratories had been transformed

into offices for the faculty members. Some of these offices were used as private outpatient clinics. This also had to stop immediately. In productive research laboratories
every inch of space is utilized for the execution of experiments. Having this in mind, I
allocated some space in the laboratory as an office for faculty members, while the rest
of the laboratory was transformed into research labs. Three laboratories previously
used for the nuclear medicine section, but non-operational for many years, were allocated for cellular and immunopathology research. A good-size laboratory space was
made available for immunochemical studies, while another room was transformed
into a "cold" room where reagents and human material were to be stored. There
was also a room where all the big centrifuges were located, and another room was
transformed into an office where the medical records of patients with autoimmune
rheumatic disease would be kept. The hematology and endocrinology laboratories
would continue their diagnostic work as before.

Neither of the two faculty members in physics had any responsibilities. So I
suggested to one of them that he move to the medical physics department of our
medical school. He accepted my proposal with pleasure. The other physics faculty
member happily became my assistant administrator. She handled all the orders
for new instruments and reagents as well as donations from grateful patients and
foundations, and unrestricted grants from the pharmaceutical industry.

Pretty soon, the pathophysiology laboratory ceased to be a dark, depressing place
and was full of life. As was mentioned previously, Dr. Fotini Skopouli undertook the
organization of the immunopathology laboratory with Dr. Menelaus Manoussakis,
who was still in rheumatology training, as her assistant. Drs. Athanasios Tzioufas
and Panayiotis Vlachoyiannopoulos took over the immunochemistry laboratory, and
had to supervise the work of six Ph.D. candidates who had come with us from
the Ioannina immunology laboratory. Drs. Tzioufas and Vlachoyiannopoulos also
assumed the responsibility for the outpatient autoimmune rheumatic disease clinic,
which was soon transformed into a center of excellence for the diagnosis and therapy
of these disorders.

The other initiative I undertook, together with the Director and Professor of
Biochemistry, Kostas Sekeris, was to organize regular scientific meetings where the
researchers in all the laboratories in the building (physiology, biochemistry, pharmacology, and pathophysiology) would make alternate presentations of their research
work. These meetings would have, as per our intentions, two goals: first, they would
provide an opportunity for researchers working in related scientific fields to create
joint research programs, and second, a critical mass of scientists would be formed
who could more effectively help their younger colleagues form a scientific point of
view.

This proposal of ours encountered strong opposition, both overt and covert,
from the professor of pharmacology. He went around the neighborhood of Goudi
(where the premises of Athens University Medical School were located)—it seems
he had nothing better to do—trying to undermine our efforts. He would say to the
older professors that these newly elected professors came here and used the excuse
of a scientific meeting to try and put us under their thumb. As a result, no one

from the pharmacology department took part in our meetings, and the participation of researchers from the other laboratories was quite limited. So our attempt at collaboration soon ground to a halt.

In closing these few lines about my first experiences in the pathophysiology clinical service and research laboratory, I would like to mention two individuals whose support helped modernize our laboratory.

My cousin, Giorgos Moutsopoulos, was serving at the time as general secretary for the peripheral region of Thessaly. He visited me at my office, at the Athens University Medical School, and noticed that the lab and the clinical service had only three telephone lines between them, all located in the professor's office. Without saying a word, he sent his friend Mr. Tsagkarestos, the representative of a telephone center company, to our hospital. Within a short time, our department had acquired a super-modern telephone center. This was the first donation to our laboratory.

The second important contributor to the modernization of our laboratory was Loukas Georgiadis, the general manager of the Greek branch of Schering-Plough. He was from Ioannina, like me. He most kindly and politely declared his readiness to help us. His contribution was like manna from heaven for us, seeing as our cash till, that is, the special account for research funding for our laboratory at the university, was still empty. He donated to our laboratory a top-quality photocopy machine, fax machines, and computers. And that's how we got started.

6.5   The Development of a Biomedical Institute in Ioannina

The basic medical sciences' departments of Ioannina University Medical School were very active in the production of new knowledge and the nurture of young researchers eager to continue their carrier in the academic field. The development of a Biomedical Research Center that would be affiliated with the Medical School was mandatory.

In 1994, while I was already a Professor at Athens University Medical School, I got a call from my friend, the Rector of the University of Ioannina, Professor Dimitrios Glaros, who asked me if I was willing to prepare along with the Professor of Cardiology of the Medical School of Ioannina, Dimitrios Sideris, a proposal for the creation of a Research Biomedical Center, in Ioannina. This proposal was planned to be submitted to the Research and Technology General Secretariat for approval. Despite the heavy workload I had undertaken to modernize the department of Pathophysiology, I accepted to carry out this task. I felt that the Medical School of Ioannina was like my own child and I was ready to struggle for its maturation and further development. In a relatively short time, the proposal for the creation of a Research Biomedical Center in Ioannina had been prepared and was submitted to the General Secretariat for Research. The Secretary General for Research, at that time, was Professor Nikos Christodoulakis. He was a smart, knowledgeable, and decisive man. We met with him several times. In fact, we presented to him our written suggestions regarding the human resources' plan, the availability of building space, and the productivity of permanent and temporary staff which would be the initial staff of the Biomedical Center. We tried to convince him of the necessity to develop such a Biomedical Center in the geographically isolated Epirus, an area that was ideal for research. He was opposed to the creation of a Biomedical Center consisting of three Institutes, but he was agreeable to the creation of a Biomedical Institute. He promised that if the evaluation of the Institute's productivity, after five years of function, could prove its success, he would give his consent to its expansion to a center with two supplementary Institutes.

One year later, with the decision of the Research and Technology Secretariat, the project of the "Institute of Biomedical Research of Ioannina" was actualized. The institute was housed in a prefab building, previously housing a University's department that was now located in a new edifice. The initial funding granted to the Institute by the government was fairly high. If I remember, the amount was around 500,000 euros. I was appointed as a vice chairman of the Board of Directors. Despite the distance and my inelastic medical and administrative responsibilities, I actively participated in the functions of the Board.

However, Greek practices such as hiring relatives without transparent procedures, and purchasing instruments that were stacked in the corridor of a prefabric building without using them, grew my worries. I didn't want to be accused of abetting obscure procedures. I was wondering if I should continue to participate in the Board. The decision to resign from the Board of Directors was triggered some years later, when the chairman of the Board, suggested, and his suggestion was supported by the Secretariat General, that the Institute should lose its independency and become part of the Foundation of Technology and Research, which was located in Heraklion, on Crete. I must confess that my fears didn't influence the prosperity of the Institute.

Today, after 23 years of function, this Institute hosts worldwide known researchers, who produce recognizable scientific work. I hope and wish that the authorities of the Research and Technology General Secretariat, after an objective assessment, would decide to transform it into a Biomedical Center which will comprise cutting-edge scientific disciplines such as Immunology, Genomics, and Biotechnology.

6.6   The Unraveling of the Department of Internal Medicine in Ioannina

The clinical, administrative, educational, and supervisory demands of my new department in Athens did not take away my interest in the performance and progress of the department of Internal Medicine that I had developed in Ioannina. After I resigned from the Ioannina University Medical School, the professor of cardiology took over my job as chairman of the internal medicine department. He was a person with a soft personality, not fond of administrative responsibilities, and primarily interested in the development of the cardiology specialty he was directing. Despite the fact that he came to Ioannina from an excellently working department of medicine in the

Athens University Medical School, during his chairmanship he allowed the complete disintegration of the internal medicine department in Ioannina. This news was quite depressing, but I could do nothing to change things around. I felt like a pater familias observing the disintegration of his family after his departure. I did, however, have at least some responsibility for the department's breakdown.

Several years prior to my departure from the Ioannina University Medical School, I was convinced by the head of the pulmonology section, who was promoted to professor, to permit the separation of his section from the internal medicine department. He based his argument on the fact that, in all other hospitals in Greece, the pulmonology sections were independent. Thus, I allowed, on paper only, the separation of his section from the department of Internal Medicine. The combined postgraduate program between his section and our department continued, however, and the residents in pulmonology were periodically rotated with trainees in the internal medicine department as well as in the emergency room. In this way, their knowledge and abilities in internal medicine were kept up to date.

After my departure from Ioannina, the second section of medicine to become independent from the department of Internal Medicine was cardiology. The chairman of the department of Internal Medicine and the head of cardiology, further promoted the model of independent sections for each medical specialty, by implying the existence of loose administrative bonds between these two medical sections. Soon afterward, the heads of the rest of the medical specialties also requested independence. Small, specialized sections were created, primarily to satisfy the ambitions of the professor-director of a specialty, rather than to serve the needs of patients, or to advance the education of the younger generation of physicians. Each section followed its own educational program. The exchange of opinions on difficult cases was abandoned. Research collaborations among physicians of different sections became a rare phenomenon.

The break-up of the internal medicine department into specialized sections is now a reality in almost all hospitals in the country. As a result, specialized sections, such as hematology, endocrinology, cardiology, pulmonology, rheumatology etc., no longer cooperate in patient care or in physician's education. This splintering of internal medicine specialties into isolated sections severely limits the exposure of physicians to a large range of diseases, and deprives the patients of effective diagnosis and treatment for their illnesses, while also encumbering the government budget, which pays for the resultant losses. It seems that the health system in our country has developed as a means of serving the doctors themselves rather than society at large.

Some departments of medicine, however, continue to function with all medical specialties. One of these is the department of Pathophysiology at the Athens University Medical School. For how long it will continue to operate as an old-style department I cannot say. Usually when the specialists reach the professorial level, at that time independence is requested.

6.7   Patience and Persistence Get Things Done

The pathophysiology post-graduate program covered the needs of both young and mature physicians in the department. It was aimed primarily at improving their clinical and diagnostic skills. Hour-long clinical pathology conferences were held every Monday and every third Thursday of each month, during which a complicated case was presented and discussed by a faculty member who was a specialist in the field. On the first and last Thursday of every month, we had an invited professor from a different medical school or another hospital. The visiting professor presented the clinical or basic research activities of his or her team. Finally, to help doctoral candidates gain experience as researchers and speakers, every Wednesday a graduate student did a critical analysis of the literature in his area of research, and a presentation of the goal, the methodology, and the progress of his experiments and their results. Through the comments and suggestions of the more senior scientists during these presentations, the graduate students furthered and improved their own research studies. Our post-graduate sessions were popular, and the classroom was always packed with young and senior colleagues (Photo 6.2).

In Athens, there are research institutes that, like us, study physiology and the pathophysiology of the immune system. We invited research teams from these institutes to actively take part in our seminars. Their participation led to scientific collaborations. At that time, during the decade of the 1990s, the law did not allow researchers from biomedical institutes to supervise, or take part in the committees overseeing the progress of post-graduate students' research toward their doctoral theses. So, unavoidably, only medical school faculty members could oversee the progress of doctoral students working in another scientific capacity. Quite often, in fact, the area of expertise of the medical school faculty member formally supervising a thesis was far removed from the research being conducted by the doctoral candidate.

Doctoral candidates from the immunology laboratories of the Pasteur Institute and the immunology laboratories of the Alexander Fleming Biomedical Sciences Research Center were among the first post-graduate students who were overseen by members of the pathophysiology faculty. The typical arrangement in these cases,

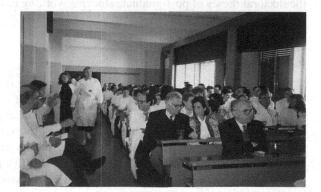

Photo 6.2 Our conference room during a seminar, packed with senior and junior faculty members, residents and Ph.D. candidates

that is, the supervision of the post-doctoral student by scientists, who were generally not well informed about the subject being studied, was not to our satisfaction. We wanted the supervisor of a doctoral thesis to be someone doing research in a related scientific area.

I put these ideas into a proposal and submitted them to the Athens University Medical School. I suggested that the supervisor, as well as the members of the advisory committee, should be researchers from various biomedical institutes in the Athens area, under whose supervision the post-graduate students would prepare their doctoral theses. I thought that this proposal was logical and scientifically sound, and I believed that I would convince my colleagues in the medical school to implement it.

In the general assembly meeting where I presented this proposal the discussions were stormy. Negative reactions from the members of the faculty could be heard everywhere: "What role will we play if we don't participate in overseeing doctoral theses?" "How can researchers who are not physicians be supervisors of medical school theses?" I tried to get across to them that the participation of researchers from institutes in the doctoral thesis committees would enhance the quality of doctoral theses, and that this would result in increasing, at no cost, the number and the caliber of medical students. My explanations went unheeded. The most extreme reactions came from the members of the junior faculty, who had been serving for many years in the Athens University Medical School. Those individuals were not familiar with how medical schools in advanced countries were run, nor had they participated in research studies. Because of this, it was difficult for them to accept my innovative proposal. Hence, the proposal was rejected with great fanfare.

Times change, however. Five years later, under a law on research, the proposal I had unsuccessfully submitted to the medical school was unanimously adopted. To put it more simply, a provision of that law designated that "researchers from institutes were allowed to supervise post-graduate students who had worked on their doctoral theses in the laboratories of the same institute."

As the years passed, I began to understand that in our country it takes a lot of time, patience, and persistence to implement reforms and bring about change. As soon as the new law was published, researchers at biomedical institutes began supervising the doctoral theses of post-graduate students working in their laboratories.

6.8 Medical Councils

In our country, there is one anachronistic practice that is still prevalent: the convocation of a medical council or joint consultation of experts to solve difficult-to-diagnose-and-treat medical problems or, in actuality, to compartmentalize medical responsibility when the patient is well known. This practice was carried over from older times when there were no specialized doctors. The participants in these councils or consultations are generally high-profile professors and physicians who are friends of the patient's family. More often than not, however, their field of expertise has little or nothing to do with the medical problem that needs to be addressed.

At these councils, the patient's own doctor presents his or her medical problems to a circle of assembled physicians, behind closed doors, in an office. Rarely does one of the participants examine the patient, but all attendees express an opinion based on what they have heard, and they leave the council after bringing the relatives up-to-date. Always with their pockets fuller than they were before they arrived. Generally, these councils offer little toward the diagnosis or treatment of the patient, but they serve to reassure the relatives, who feel that they have done everything possible for their loved one.

From my first years back in Greece, I refused to participate in such councils. But I always offered my help when I was asked to visit a patient in a hospital in Athens or Thessaloniki. Generally, it was for cases within my field of knowledge, that is, diseases that were due to an attack on bodily organs by the immune system. Many of these cases are still very vivid in my memory.

When I assumed the post of chairman of the pathophysiology department in Athens, I was summoned by a senior professor of internal medicine to participate in one such council. I was ashamed to refuse to participate, when the other participants were all professors of internal medicine at the Athens University Medical School.

I will not tire you with the details and the problems of the patient in question. I will simply say that the specific medical problem was in my special field of knowledge. I asked the chairman of the department to allow me to examine the patient. He reluctantly agreed. After examining the patient, I asked the professor of internal medicine in attendance, who was a hematologist, to examine the patient's blood smear himself. After he gave us his opinion, I presented to the colleagues in attendance the diagnosis of the patient's disorder and recommended the proper course of treatment. It was a rare disorder and the complications in the case of that patient had not been described before in any international medical journal. But I had a similar case in my department. The material from those two cases formed the basis for the publication of an article.

The time came for the briefing of the patient's relatives, and this happened as it usually does in these medical councils. I thought that my role was over and I was preparing to leave. All of a sudden, the door opened and a young colleague came into the office holding up a fistful of closely pressed envelopes like an open hand of cards. He began distributing them, starting from the senior professor. When my turn came, I asked him for his name and his position in the hospital. He answered that he was a resident. The fact that a resident, instead of attending the council and learning something from his teachers, was performing the function of a money distributor disturbed me deeply. Without showing the customary respect for my senior colleagues, I told him how I felt. Everyone froze. I did not accept my envelope, and I exited the office leaving everyone surprised at my reaction.

The story of what my colleagues saw as my ill-mannered actions soon circulated in and around Athens. From that time on, I have never been invited to a medical council. I am now spared from that oppressive, meaningless procedure. Very often, however, I am asked for my opinion by colleagues in many hospitals in Athens, and I always give it freely. I believed, and still do, that a functionary of the State Healthcare System has no right to be paid extra for his opinion by a patient being treated in a state hospital.

6.9   The Scourge of Medical Schools and the Healthcare System

6.9.1   Nepotism and Internal Favoritism

Greek physicians seeking a better education, after their graduation from medical school, emigrate to Europe, the U.S., and even to the Far East to acquire knowledge and improve their professional skills. Those with drive, passion, and dedication involve themselves in research, discover its beauty, produce new medical knowledge, and attain high-level academic or research posts. But are the medical schools in Greece willing or able to attract them? Unfortunately, anachronistic practices such as nepotism and what can here be called "internal favoritism," keep the doors of our medical schools hermetically sealed to outsiders.

Nepotism is the inheritance of a powerful person's profession or position by a descendant or a relative. Of course it is easy to understand how a physician can, through his example, pass on to his children the attractions, challenges, difficulties and rewards of the medical profession. On the other hand, it is difficult to comprehend the machinations through which democratic processes enable the heirs of current or retired university professors to acquire a faculty position at a medical school. It should not be overlooked, however, that some university offspring, unfortunately, the minority, are well educated and prepared enough to deserve an advertised university position. This, however, is not the rule. Usually, professorial positions, when planned for a poorly qualified relative of a professor, are announced cut to fit the relative's qualifications, and the rank and appointments committee is selected for that purpose. In this way more capable candidates are excluded from the process, and the position is granted to a professor's heir.

A study was performed on faculty members of randomly selected clinical or laboratory departments from the Athens University Medical School to substantiate this allegation. A questionnaire was given to them asking about the profession of their parents. The results were striking. The survey showed that 55% of 140 former or active professors of the medical school helped a relative become a faculty member of the medical school. In other words, the probability of a professor's relative becoming a faculty member was 2:1. By contrast, the possibility of offspring of parents (around 300,000) with jobs unrelated to medical school becoming faculty members was from $3/10^3$ to $3/10^4$. To make a long story short, nepotism in our medical schools is thriving. The university, however, is not the only Greek institution in which nepotism is prevalent. The same picture can be seen in the parliament. In fact, members of the same three families have been governing Greece for the last seventy years.

The other detrimental factor keeping our medical schools back from international recognition is internal favoritism or the occupation of high-ranking professorial posts through the promotion of lower-ranking faculty members already working in the school. This practice does not favor the enrichment of the faculty body with new members with contemporary ideas, knowledge, and advanced professional skills. Why then does this practice prevail? Probably because some faculty members, perhaps with low academic credentials, promote colleagues and friends, with the sole purpose of consolidating their own power within the medical school. It appears that they are fearful of colleagues with superior qualities. In this way, mediocrity breeds mediocrity.

Let's consider the following blatant example of internal favoritism: a relatively young Greek university professor, in his late forties, from a prominent U.S. medical school, with an impressive curriculum vitae, after twenty years abroad, wants to return home. A professorial post in his field of specialization is announced. With enthusiasm the professor from the U.S. decides to apply for the job.

Scene one: A relative of the candidate calls the school to find out what the necessary papers for the application are. Instead of providing the information, the school administrator gives a brazen, incontestable response: "This position is for Dr. So-and-So, who is already a faculty member in our school." In other words, the administrator unabashedly declares that the legal procedure is just a formality. The position has already been given.

Scene two: Despite the warning, the professorial candidate applies for the job. After some days, he receives a message from a professor in the Greek medical school, saying he wants to talk to him. The professorial candidate calls him. "Hello, I am Mr. So-and-So." Oh, yes, I remember you from your student years," the professor of the Greek university replies, and continues: "It was obvious from your student days that you would become a researcher and an academic. But why did you apply for the job of professor without asking us? This position is for So-and-So." The candidate does not leave the illegal statement unanswered: "The announcement of the position called for everyone with qualifications to apply. The position was open to everyone with the proper credentials." Without hesitation, the professor gives an entirely unacademic answer: "I just want to warn you that if you insist on going forward with this candidacy, you will pay for this in any future attempts to be elected professor in Greece." Statements like this from a university professor smack of a favor-swapping, horse-trading mentality.

Scene three: The professorial candidate does not withdraw his candidacy. He visits the chairman of the department to see what he has to say. Instead of asking the candidate what his plans are for advancing his specialty in the school, what space he needs for his research work, where he will apply for grants to support his work, how much time he will allocate for students' education, he too makes some very un-academic remarks. The chairman blatantly tells the candidate: "You have a very good academic background and have done remarkable research work. However, we are not interested in hiring research-oriented faculty members." And he continues, "We might announce an associate professor position for you in the future if you withdraw your candidacy now." The professorial candidate feels compelled to answer the other's comments and suggestions: "With all due respect, I'm surprised to hear that you are not interested in hiring faculty members with a solid research background. Without research the international recognition of your school will be extremely poor. And what's more, I didn't declare my candidacy to horse-trade, but to be judged impartially on the basis of my qualifications." The chairman loses his temper. It seems he is accustomed to servile behavior, to people playing up to him and flattering him, not judging him. Professors like these who have crawled their way to the top without qualifications often seem to have inflated egos and believe they are untouchable and can say whatever comes into their mind without caring at all about the School's wellbeing.

If a periodic, objective evaluation of all faculty members was a rule in our University Schools, individuals without academic ethics, or the ability to generate and communicate new knowledge and to convey professional and moral values would be forced to leave the Schools.

It does not require hard thinking to guess who was elected to the advertised professorial post! Needless to say, it was the "internally favored" candidate, the one without academic credentials.

Nepotism and internal favoritism are among the major factors that lead to the proliferation of faculty members with mediocre academic records. Fortunately, there are some foci of excellence in Greek medical schools that still attract well-trained individuals as faculty members, produce high-quality academic work, and contribute to a medical school's good reputation.

6.9.2   How to Deal with "Black Money"

"Black money" is known in Greece as a "fakellaki," a word that refers to the "envelope" in which such money is delivered. Among the public services where this practice still thrives are the country's hospitals. While we natives have first-hand experience with this practice, international organizations, such as the OECD, have analyzed it from time to time in their reports. The insertion of "black money" into a professional, non-monetary relationship degrades the physician's professional status, undervalues the personality of the patient, and is a serious source of income loss for the state.

In order to deal with this phenomenon, we must first make some necessary distinctions so as to acquire a better sense of what goes on. There are indeed some corrupt doctors in public hospitals, who take advantage of weak or needy patients by demanding and accepting under-the-table payments for medical services that should have been offered for free. This practice is a criminal offense, and it is the duty of medical associations to expel corrupt colleagues from their ranks.

Within the public health system, private transactions between the patient and the doctor still flourish because they are accepted by both parties. The patient often chooses a physician because of his or her reputation. This "private" patient is treated as a special case and given priority both for treatment and a bed in a privileged hospital room. After the successful solution of his medical problems, the patient feels obliged to compensate the physician for his services. This transaction can involve from a few hundred to a few thousand euros. All this occurs while the hospital administration turns a blind eye. It amounts to a crypto-privatization of the public health system which, leaving aside the moral dimension of the issue, leads to multiple financial losses. First, the patient cannot deduct the expense from his taxable income. Second, the state does not collect the corresponding tax. And third, the hospital, while providing the material and technical infrastructure for the patient's therapeutic, medical, and nursing care as well as administrative staff, is not compensated by the substantial "private" doctor-patient relationship.

It is naïve to think that this mentality can only be tackled by oppressive measures. This mentality has many causes. It starts with the fact that patient X seeks the medical services of physician Y, usually one of the best-qualified physicians in the public health system. And then there are the unacceptably low salaries of the medical staff at public hospitals in relation to the quality and the quantity of work they provide. This fact encourages some physicians to engage in opaque transactions. A third essential cause of this third-world behavior is the state's theoretical obsession that public health services are "free," which makes its representatives in the hospital administration prone to ignoring violations involving money. Finally, these illegal practices are tolerated by the mismanaged administrations of hospitals which, as a rule, are run by party members or former officials without education and experience in hospital administration.

How can this practice be abolished? We do not need to reinvent the wheel. Others have already done this. Quite simply, the "private" physician–patient relationship, instead of being conducted in secret, should be done openly and transparently through the official system of the hospital. In this way, through private operations in public hospitals, the incomes of the physicians will increase, the state will enjoy the corresponding taxes when this income is declared, and the hospital will have an additional source of revenue to help modernize its infrastructure. This mixed mode of operation in public hospitals has been adopted in the oldest public health system in Europe, that of Great Britain, as well as in the Netherlands and in Germany. Why not imitate them?

It goes without saying that this mixed mode of operation should not deny good medical care to needy patients, who are not able to compensate the physician. These individuals should be treated equally with those who can afford to pay. To achieve this delicate balance, physicians in public hospitals should not be allowed to treat "privately" more than a certain percentage of patients out of the total number they treat each month. In order for such a practice to be successfully implemented, it is of paramount importance that ingrained pathologies in our country, such as tax evasion, be eradicated.

6.10   The Predictions of a Palm Reader

The reader may remember that one night back in the spring of 1977, while returning home from Cafritz Memorial Hospital after my evening shift in the emergency room, I visited a famous palm reader. After studying my palm, she predicted all the important events in my life.

It was now 1999, and the sudden onset of a serious medical problem brought back to my mind those twenty-year-old predictions:

Prediction 1: You will divorce.

Indeed after ten years of married life, Lambrini and I could not make our marriage work, and despite the fact that we had two very young, wonderful children, whom we both loved, our lives took different directions.

Prediction 2: In the middle of your life you will become seriously ill, but you will survive.

In fact, at the age of fifty-five, I was returning from Vienna after giving a talk at a scientific meeting there. After my talk, I felt a heavy pressure in my chest. I didn't say anything to my colleagues. I took an aspirin and a nitroglycerine sublingual pill and the symptoms subsided. I didn't join my colleagues at the prearranged meeting. The next morning I took the airplane to return home. The nagging pain in my chest continued. Upon my arrival I went straight to the hospital and I was admitted to the coronary care unit. Thinking back on the unsophisticated steps I took for my condition, I was lucky I didn't die. Coronary angiography revealed a serious atherosclerotic lesion on my main coronary artery. Without delay, I was taken to the operating room and a successful bypass surgery was performed. My rehabilitation kept me out of work for approximately one month, during which time I continued to closely monitor my colleagues' research. I remembered that palm reader's predictions, as I tried to determine why I developed an atherosclerotic lesion at such a young age. There were many contributing factors. First was my heavy smoking habit. Second, the lack of exercise. Third, the continuous stress in my professional life as I clashed with colleagues in order to accomplish my often unreachable goals; and finally, my autoimmune background, since autoimmune reactivity plays a significant role in the pathogenesis of atherosclerosis. Obviously, this major health event was a wake-up call for me and, with the help of Fotini, I changed my lifestyle completely. I quit smoking and for a prolonged period of time I followed a strict exercise program. After this life-changing event, I returned stronger and more determined than ever to my work, and some months later I undertook yet another responsibility: the chairmanship of the National Organization for Medicines in parallel with the chairmanship of the department of Pathophysiology at the Athens University Medical School.

Prediction 3: You will reach the top of your profession.

I can say, in all modesty, that she was right about that too.

6.11 Public Official: National Policy for Medicines

6.11.1 First Period: President, National Committee for a List of Prescription Medicines

As a professional practicing medicine in Greece, there were many things that troubled my medical conscience. One practice in particular was extremely annoying. Many colleagues prescribed medications with little or no therapeutic value. People would show up at our outpatient clinic holding a fistful of medications that by and large contained no therapeutic ingredients. I would try to encourage them to discontinue medications with no therapeutic efficacy and are possibly harmful to their system. My suggestions, however, had little or no influence on the practices of colleagues. The pharmaceutical industry had many ways to endorse the use of these placebo-like medications.

In the mid-1980s, the then Vice-Minister of Social Security, Dr. Grigoris Solomos, tried to confront the uncalled-for prescribing of pharmaceutical substances by doctors working for the state social security administration (known by its acronym IKA), by appointing a committee for the listing of prescription medicines based on evidence. He included me in that committee. The position of the committee's president was given to a professor of pharmacology who, in addition to his academic post, was also serving as an advisor to pharmaceutical companies. Unfortunately, this conflict of interest had not been taken into account before appointing him president of the committee. From the very first meeting of the committee, it was clear as day that his goal was to curtail the committee's functioning.

In his opening address he reminded the members of the committee that a licensed medical physician had the freedom to prescribe, according to his judgement, any medications that were licensed to circulate by the National Organization for Medicines. In his speech, he neglected to mention, perhaps deliberately, that many of the medications in circulation had no demonstrated therapeutic benefit and were quite possibly harmful to those using them, while it is certain that they made the prescribing physicians and the pharmaceutical company richer. For every useless or unnecessary medication physicians prescribed, they were reimbursed, in one way or another, by the pharmaceutical industry.

The president of the Committee for a List of Prescription Medications functioned more like a guardian angel for pharmaceutical companies than a protector of patients' health. His influence was strong, and the power newly conferred on him substantial, and because of this, the committee itself was short-lived. The attempt to bring pharmaceuticals up-to-date in our country died while it was still in its infancy.

Many years later, in the spring of 1996, the government under Costas Simitis decided to put some order in the pharmaceutical sector. They sincerely wanted to create a list of prescription medicines. I received a phone call from the then Vice-Minister of Health, Dr. Nikolaos Farmakis, a classmate of mine in medical school, and he asked me if I would take on that difficult, thorny task. He was familiar with all the problems facing the pharmaceutical sector in our country, and he wanted to put some order there in any way he could. I conveyed to him my reservations, since I was well acquainted with the evil networks of the pharmaceutical industry, but he very convincingly assured me that they were determined to "root out the evil down to the bone" and that "they had every intention of vigorously supporting my actions toward this end." After many meetings, a committee of specialists was appointed for the establishment of a National List of Prescription Medicines.

What exactly is this list and what is its purpose? It is a list of pharmaceutical substances that is determined by a committee of specialists, based on strictly scientific and economic criteria. Its purpose is to protect public health through the prescription of safe medications, whose efficacy has been verified by double-blind studies, and at the same time to reduce public pharmaceutical expenses by excluding ineffective pharmaceutical substances from the National List of Prescription Medicines.

This list must be constantly updated because every day new safe and effective pharmaceutical substances are being produced. Most European countries have such lists. It was time for our country to do the same.

I was appointed president of the committee. I took on this task with great enthusiasm, well disposed to devote time to it from the little remaining to me after my academic obligations. I was expecting an uphill battle. I don't know why, but I believed that I would be successful. Fortunately, all the members of the committee were very well educated on their subject, had impeccable moral credentials, and were keen to create a list. We all believed that every patient in our country had the right to proper treatment with the use of medications whose benefits were proven. In this way, with the rational and strictly scientific compilation of the list, medicine overuse would be effectively curbed, public health would be protected, the imprudent waste of public money would be kept in check, and the health of our citizens would not be threatened in the least.

There are two more compelling reasons for the creation of a list in our country:

(a) In order for a pharmaceutical substance to circulate commercially it must go through an assiduous, painstaking, scientific examination as to its efficacy and safety. This procedure is carried out by the National Organization of Medicines. In our country, as is the case for other similar procedures, the examination of medicines, before a license to circulate is granted, was frequently conducted in a haphazard way, and often the criteria used had less to do with science and more to do with the pharmaceutical industry.

(b) In the pharmaceutical market, aside from the originally produced pharmaceutical substances, there were also generic versions in circulation. Generic medications are cheaper than the originals and help the economy of the country. Granting them a license, however, requires the same strict controls as are used for the originals.

After many hours of discussion in the committee, we set out the basic principles for the creation of the list:

(1) Substances would be included in the list, if they were already licensed and circulating in three or more of the following countries: England, France, Germany, Sweden, Switzerland, and the United States.

(2) For the remaining pharmaceutical substances that did not have a license to circulate in the above-mentioned countries, a thorough search of the medical literature would be performed, and the substances chosen would be those with the best efficacy and safety records, as shown and substantiated by research studies published in reputable scientific journals.

(3) The generic pharmaceutical substances would be included in the list if their price did not exceed the average daily cost of treatment provided by the original pharmaceutical preparations.

Through the application of these criteria, plus a year and a half of hard work, the list of prescription medicines became a reality. We submitted the list to the Ministry of Social Security and Health and to the Hellenic Association of Pharmaceutical Companies for their comments. We held a press conference with the relevant vice-ministers to explain to the Greek people the reasons for the creation of the list and assure them that this would not deny them access to medicines with therapeutic benefits.

My impressions from this interview were deeply disturbing. The journalists' questions seemed to me to have a purpose other than serving the interests of the Greek people. Their focus seemed to be geared toward the pharmaceutical industry. Needless to say, the list disturbed well-established interests, either because it did not include useless medicines, or because it excluded generic versions of medicines that were more expensive than the originals.

After the interview, there was a rash of articles against the list in the press, which resulted, as was probably their goal, in creating feelings of confusion and insecurity in people. Those articles were purportedly based on the opinions of "renowned specialists," who claimed that the list marginalized important therapeutic substances. The vested interests aligned against the establishment of a National List of Medicines, taking advantage of the confusion that they themselves had created, convinced those in charge of the two relevant ministries and the then-serving president of the National Organization for Medicines, that the list was completely unfair to the Greek pharmaceutical industry, seeing as a sizeable number of their products had not been included in the list. They managed to arrange a meeting that would be attended by the relevant vice-ministers, the president of the National Organization for Medicines, a representative of the pharmaceutical industry, and me. At this meeting, they claimed, they would prove that a great injustice had been done.

We met at the office of the vice-minister of Social Security. The representative of the pharmaceutical industry turned to me with a forlorn expression and said: "My dear professor, with the list you have created two hundred Greek families will be out of work." I solemnly answered him: "I believe the list we have created protects the health of all ten million Greeks." My answer was not well received. It was clear that their criteria for the eligibility of medicines were not the same as ours and not strictly scientific. In fact, they did not even serve society at large but simply their own self-interests. They were trying to protect their own economic interests under the cloak of the supposed unemployment that would be caused by the list.

I must also say here that, in order to prove his point, he handed me ten reprints of articles that he believed proved that the medicines we had rejected were scientifically appropriate. The articles were all from Greek magazines and were lacking, I am sorry to say, any kind of scientific documentation. I pointed this out immediately, noting that the requirements for the inclusion of a pharmaceutical substance in the list specify that its efficacy and safety be proven by studies published in reputable international journals. The articles that were given to me could not stand up to even the slightest analysis or criticism. They were only useful to people, who were not able to evaluate scientific studies. In front of everyone I tossed the articles they gave me into the wastepaper basket. "What are you doing?", he said to me. "Don't you realize that you are insulting your colleagues?" "I am not insulting anyone," I answered. "But I can't abide unsubstantiated scientific opinions." The meeting was adjourned in a rather heavy atmosphere but, from what it seemed at least, without the opponents of the list having their way.

The pharmaceutical industry continued to strongly promote their views, both above and below the surface. The politicians in charge soon fell in line. Their first capitulation was to accept the creation of a secondary committee that would examine whether or not pharmaceutical substances had been correctly excluded from the list. The result of this was the re-inclusion in the list of some of the medicines that had been previously rejected as ineffective. The efforts of two years of hard and honest work were thereby wiped out, and a scientific and moral choice with no other goal than to protect public health and public money was invalidated. I had no other option then but to resign. I left my position as the president of the committee with my head held high, without having deviated during my tenure from the dictates of my scientific conscience, or the principles of medical ethics and my moral obligations.

Certain colleagues, supposedly fair-minded academics, celebrated my resignation through articles in the press. It appears that many such colleagues, covered by the cloak of science, serve the pharmaceutical industry more than their patients, medical truth, and the public interest. My answer to them was that the short-term implementation of the list of medicines led to a 40% reduction in pharmaceutical expenses. Unfortunately, due to a lack of statistics, it was not easy to estimate the benefits of the list to overall public health. It is not by chance, however, that in 2005, the year that the list of medicines was abolished, pharmaceutical expenses in our country increased by 100%. But what does all that matter? The then-serving minister of health who abolished the list, as was reported in the newspaper *Eleftherotypia* at the time, received financial support for his electoral campaign as an MP from a pharmaceutical company.

6.11.2 Second Period: President, National Organization for Medicines

The subject of the inadequate regulation of medicines in Greece kept coming back. Early in 1999, Dr. Nikolaos Farmakis, the Vice-Minister of Health, notified me that the government and the Prime Minister of Greece, Costas Simitis, were again anxious to put some order in what is often referred to here in Greece as the "evil pharmaceutical circuits." This time they offered me the presidency of the National Organization for Medicines. My unpleasant experience with the list made me reluctant to assume the post I was offered. I thanked them for the honor but said that I wanted some time to think things over and decide whether or not I wanted to take on the job. In essence, I did not want to waste my time without being certain that I had something to offer. I was not at all sure, in spite of the assurances of complete government support, that the pharmaceutical circuits could be defeated. The government officials sincerely assured me that they would support any and every action of mine whose goal was to reform pharmaceutical distribution and that my decisions as president of the National Organization for Medicines would be fully respected by the ministry overseeing us.

This invitation kept me occupied for months. I had many meetings with the minister and vice-minister of health. I also talked with the General Secretary of the Cabinet, Socrates Kosmidis. He was the inspiration behind the attempt to regulate pharmaceutical distribution, and it was he who implemented the drastic and impressive reduction of drug prices toward the end of 1997. I was impressed by his extensive knowledge of the problems in the pharmaceutical sector in Greece, and also by the seriousness of his outlook and his unshakeable conviction that the public health sector in our country needed to be modernized. "We have to fight for this," he said. He assured me that the prime minister would be an avid supporter of whatever we did. In an attempt to politely avoid the unpleasant consequences and possible failure of these efforts, I asked the government ministers for various guarantees, hoping that they would not be given. For example, I asked that the board of directors of the organization would not include members of unions or political groups. I also asked that the board of directors be comprised of scientists whose fields of study were related to the medications the organization was overseeing. They accepted all my proposals and, in fact, improved on them. They asked that I be the one to propose the scientists I believed had the proper moral values and scientific capabilities to function as members of the board of directors of the organization.

The other thing I asked for was that the presidency at the organization would not disrupt my work as the chairman of the department of Pathophysiology at the Athens University Medical School. We had by then, after six years of hard work, created an optimally functioning university department and a research laboratory that was producing innovative medical knowledge. I did not want to leave the directorship of the department. My colleagues, although their scientific abilities and ethics were excellent, had not yet acquired the expertise to run a university department as large as ours had become. In other words, I asked for my post as president of the National Organization for Medicines to be unpaid and part-time. The legal department of the Ministry of Health and the Cabinet responded that my request was reasonable, would not create any legal problems, and that they would honor it. The acceptance of all my demands convinced me that the government did indeed want to correct the shortcomings in the pharmaceutical sector, and also canceled out the excuses and objections I had put forward.

In September, 1999, I assumed the presidency of the National Organization for Medicines. The Vice-President, Dr. T. Kefalas, a pharmacologist who had already been serving the organization for many years, remained in his position. He was a man of high moral caliber, a tireless worker well acquainted with the problems that had been besieging the pharmaceutical sector in our country, easy to work with, and low-key. After many meetings, we set out the initial and urgent goals for the improvement of the functioning of the organization:

- Complete transparency in all our actions.
- Increasing the number and caliber of outside scientists to evaluate the safety and efficacy of new pharmaceutical substances, and the application of higher-quality criteria to select them.
- Speeding up the procedure for evaluating all products whose approval was still pending.
- Strict implementation of the regulation to deny membership on the board of directors of the organization to in-house and outside employees in the event of a conflict of interest.
- Weekly monitoring of the operation of the administration of the organization, with a meeting every Friday of the president and the vice-president with the section directors of the organization.
- Frequent and thorough updating of health professionals concerning: (a) new, safe and effective pharmaceutical products, and (b) the side effects observed from pharmaceutical substances already licensed to circulate. For this purpose, the scientific journal of the Pan-Hellenic Medical Association *Iatriko Vima* allowed us a page in every issue for "News from the National Organization for Medicines."

We conveyed these initial goals to the board of directors. They were unanimously accepted. During my many long years of service in Greece I was a member of many boards of directors. The Board of the National Organization for Medicines was completely free from the usual small-mindedness, self-serving and obstructionist thinking, and mental and emotional exhaustion. The meetings of the board of directors, in spite of the many subjects on the agenda, never lasted more than two hours. I always left feeling relaxed, happy, and satisfied.

Applying the rules of transparency, we informed the Hellenic Association of Pharmaceutical Companies that, from that time forward, their representatives who had issues or complaints could address them to the president and the vice-president of the National Organization for Medicines.

To reduce the pressure and possible, although forbidden, attempts by representatives of the pharmaceutical industry to influence employees at the National Organization for Medicines, we established a visitor log at the entrance to the organization, as is moreover specified by the European Medicines Agency (EMA). In this book, detailed records were kept of visits by representatives of pharmaceutical companies and the employees to whom visits were made.

To accelerate the pace of approval of new pharmaceutical substances, we increased the number of evaluators from forty to three hundred, selecting individuals of high scientific caliber and impeccable ethics. By doing this, we reduced the time needed to evaluate pharmaceutical products, and gradually and substantially brought down the number of applications for approval that had been pending for many years at the organization.

An important part of the national policy for medicines in our country is the domestic production of generic medicines. These generic copies, once their equivalence with the original medicines was established, would be less of a drain on the public coffers since they would be cheaper. In addition, the domestic production of medicines would give a boost to the country's economy.

The laboratories that study the equivalence between original and generic medicines were all privately run. It was rumored that their results were often manipulated. We had to find a scientific means of performing our assessments without the fear that the results they gave us had been falsified. After much discussion, the right person was found who could evaluate the results of the comparative bioequivalencies. It was bio-statistician Ourania Dafni, an associate professor of nursing at Athens University. A top-notch scientist with a strong sense of responsibility, she was highly intelligent and industrious.

In one of the cases that she was assigned, she noticed from the start, after measuring absorption rates of original and generic pharmaceutical substances in the gastroenterological tracts of an actual human population, that the bio-equivalency curves were exactly the same for the original and the generic copy. To obtain such similar absorption curves is simply not possible, no matter how optimally the generic copy is produced. After a thorough investigation, she confirmed the adulteration of the clinical data and revealed the algorithm that had been used to arrive at the false results. She informed me of the obvious fraud, and I instructed her to bring the matter up to the board to be dealt with legally. The generic version was not approved by the relevant primary committee. The file was then sent to a secondary committee, which upheld the verdict of the first committee, but did not make its decision known until three years later. In the meantime, I resigned and there had been many changes in the administration.

During that time, Ourania Dafni visited the National Organization for Medicines and tried to persuade the administration to take legal action against the clearly evident fraud. Unfortunately, this resulted in the poor lady being accused in turn. And here is why. The company that had evaluated the pharmaceutical equivalencies filed a lawsuit against Ourania Dafni supposedly for libel. So, she found herself in the position of the accused for having sworn under oath to try and protect public health while serving the National Organization for Medicines. I testified in her defense, as did many other colleagues who rallied to her side. After many hassles and difficulties, she was acquitted by a court ruling. It was a bitter experience that stayed with her. She spent no mean sum of money on legal fees and lawyers, all for conscientiously performing her scientific and social duty.

Pharmacovigilance was another function of the organization that was seriously lacking. What exactly is pharmacovigilance? It is the recording and reporting to the National Organization of Medicines by physicians of the side effects of medicines that are licensed to circulate. The report of the adverse effects is made on a specially designed printed form, the "yellow card," which is the same for everyone. By making these reports, every physician contributes to the circulation of safe medicines throughout the population. The yellow card reports are evaluated by the National Organization for Medicines, and their assessment leads to the modification of the instructions for the usage of medicines or their withdrawal from circulation. This practice had not taken root among health professionals in our country, nor had it borne any fruit.

Studies had shown that in Greece only 3.5 mentions of adverse side effects of medicines were reported per 1,000 physicians, while in Great Britain the figure was 414 per 1,000 physicians. We had to remedy this. We needed to impress upon our colleagues, as soon as possible, the importance of collecting and reporting data on adverse side effects of drugs to the National Organization for Medicines. We planned two meetings for the academic year 1999–2000 to educate health professionals in pharmacovigilance, one in Athens and the other in Ioannina. Both were very successful. Many questions were brought up. The thing most feared by our colleagues was that perhaps by reporting side effects they would be held responsible for them, or alternately that they would give the impression of not being well informed. Through our answers we tried to put their misgivings to rest. But in order for this system to succeed, continuous updating and education are required, and I am afraid that our country is still far behind in this area.

In order to carry out the goals we had set, I spent two hours every morning at the organization, plus the entire morning on Fridays and the entire afternoon on Thursdays meeting with the board of directors.

Everyone, both friends and enemies, had to admit that there was something new in the wind. But the wind can often bring clouds with it. The first cloud was not long in coming. Some of the employees of the organization were upset by a notice of ours specifying that they were not allowed to have meals with representatives of pharmaceutical companies, nor was it permitted for them to accept any gifts of significant value from those representatives.

An enthusiastic and combative member of parliament (MP) from the opposition party, although he was a member of the junior faculty of the medical school, seemed to not quite grasp what a conflict of interest meant, and submitted a question to the Parliament asking why the new administration of the National Organization for Medicines was terrorizing its employees. We prepared an answer to the question, which would be presented by Vice-Minister, Nikolaos Farmakis. We included in the text we gave him the rules and regulations pertaining to conflicts of interest currently in use by the European Medicines Agency. The minister's answer to the MP's question brooked no objections, and the question was sent to the trash bin.

The second cloud on the horizon, the one that would carry the storm with it, was of little interest to me, nor did I spend any time dealing with it. It was a letter published in the well-known newspaper *Kathimerini*. It was signed by an emeritus professor of pharmacology who, by coincidence, happened to be an avowed opponent of a national list of prescription medicines. The letter claimed that I had been illegally appointed president of the organization. I notified the Department of Health and the office of the secretary general of the Cabinet. They put my mind to rest and advised me not pay any attention to such publications.

I carried on with my work. Our targets, minor and major, were being met every day. After a thorough review of the organization's activities and the section directors' contributions, I was able to formulate my own view of each of them. Toward the end of 1999, I decided to do a serious reshuffling of the section heads, intended to curtail the possible illegitimate influence of third parties on the activities of the National Organization for Medicines. Everyone was stunned. They understood that I did not take my job as president lightly. It was very encouraging that there were no serious negative reactions within the organization. In outside circles, however, objections were slowly mounting among those who did not want any changes in the organization.

Early in the year 2000, I received a phone call from the rector of the university. After expressing his admiration for my achievements as the chairman of Pathophysiology, he politely said that he was "very sad" to have to inform me that the president of the medical school had forwarded him the letter published in *Kathimerini* and that he was afraid that my position as president of the organization was not legal. "I am obliged," he told me "to forward this to the Ministry of Education for their opinion." I answered that the government had assured me that my appointment was legal. I angrily told him that he ought to be dealing with the colleagues serving in our school who do not follow the rules of proper ethical conduct when practicing as physicians. He listened to me patiently, and then politely ended our conversation, but he proceeded with a series of actions that eventually led to my resignation.

The work of modernizing the organization was moving forward day by day, slowly but surely. The "News from the National Organization for Medicines" was published religiously in the journal *Iatriko Vima*. With a grant from an anonymous donor, completely unrelated to the drug industry, we prepared and printed a bilingual (Greek-English) flier that outlined the function and goals of the organization. In this way, anyone interested in the National Organization for Medicines could be kept updated. We created two new committees. The first, Science and Ethics Committee for the Approval of Clinical Studies, was led by Professor Nikos Pavlidis, and the second, Approval of Funding for Medical Conferences, by the former Vice-President of the organization, Dr. Stavros Kazazis, a pharmacologist. Prior to that time, approval for the funding of medical conferences was granted by the president of the organization.

We got rid of all personal telephone lines and the organization acquired a telephone center. We updated the way employees were paid. All employees would now have their salaries deposited directly into their bank accounts. This did away with those shameful long lines, every fifteen days, outside the organization's cashier's office. This clearly needed administrative practice took some time to implement. And why do you think that was? Because the people who had previously physically handed out the money lost their tips. We also gave incentives to the employees to be trained in the use of computers. Our goal was for the organization to operate with its own computer network. Those plans, however, remained on paper only. During my time there, at least, we did not manage to implement them.

At some point in my tenure at the National Organization for Medicines, I met a brilliant biomathematics expert, Elias Zinzaras. He was working on the evaluation of pharmaceutical products. I was surprised by the fact that a public employee was publishing scientific studies in top-rated journals. I decided at that time to upgrade the organization scientifically by extending its scope to research. The first research program evaluated the effectiveness of generic medicines, as attested by the bio-equivalency studies carried out by the National Organization for Medicines from the time I took over the organization's administration. We also decided to investigate the factors that led to increased expenses for antibiotics. This study showed that the new and expensive antibiotics were more frequently prescribed than the older and cheaper antibiotics, thus accounting for the increase in pharmaceutical expenses.

Dr. Zinzaras received permission from the organization's administration to use the archives of Farmetrika Inc. (an affiliate of the National Organization for Medicines), to evaluate how antibiotics were prescribed in different districts of Greece. The results were impressive. It was shown that in a specific district, antibiotics from one particular pharmaceutical company were prescribed, while in another district the antibiotics of another company were overprescribed. In other words, the pharmaceutical companies had divided up the pharmaceutical market for antibiotics, so that each one of them had an equal profit. The results of the study were published in the *Journal of Antimicrobial Chemotherapy*. Today, Elias Zintzaras is among the best biomathematicians in the country. He is a professor of biomathematics at the Thessaly University Medical School.

One of the three lawyers of the organization retired during my tenure. It was an opportunity for the organization to acquire a legal advisor who was familiar with the European legal system and in particular with the legal framework for medicines. After a formal proposal from me, the board of directors approved the specifications for the above qualifications for hiring a new legal advisor. Eleven candidates applied. Four of them fulfilled the requirements specified in the announcement. The committee that would select the winning candidate, based on the legal framework, was comprised of the president of the organization, the director of the organization's legal services, a representative of the Athens Bar Association, a court magistrate, and the director of the administrative department of the organization. After many delays the committee met. By that time, I had left the organization. They selected a lawyer not particularly well-suited to the post, but who had the additional qualification of being a close relative of an MP of the party then in power. Ah, the glory of Greece!

In early 2000, the term of the primary and secondary committees for the authorization of new pharmaceutical products, biological substances, pharmacovigilance, and pharmaceutical products for veterinary use expired. This was yet another opportunity to modernize the organization. The new presidents and committee members we proposed were all of the high scientific standing, irreproachable ethics, and extremely eager to offer their services. The Ministry of Health, after many meetings, finally approved our proposals.

It was now winter, 2000, and the television channels and the mass media were whipping up a storm with almost weekly coverage of dramatically portrayed new cases of meningitis seen in such-and-such a region of the country. I asked specialists on infectious diseases and epidemiology in Greece if the number of cases at that time of year was greater than the number of cases observed during the same period of the previous year. They all assured me that there was no cause for worry. During one of the meetings of our board of directors, I realized what was behind the announcements of new cases in the mass media and the panic they wanted to create.

The committee for biological products, following a proposal that was presented to the organization by Mrs. Kritikou, an unassuming, highly ethical, and meticulous employee, decided that the administration of the vaccine for meningococcus should be carried out solely by the country's health centers after it has been determined by epidemiological studies that there are increased cases of meningitis caused by the particular strain of the virus against which the vaccine was designed to protect. This proposal was unanimously adopted by the board of directors. After a proposal of my own, we went one step further. We prepared a press release saying the following: 1. The vaccine for meningococcus is not recommended for mass usage because: (a) it only protects against one particular strain of the virus, and (b) it therefore gives a false sense of security concerning protection from the virus for the population at large, and (c) it does not protect children under two years of age. 2. It should be administered by health centers only after it has been established that there are increased cases, due to the particular strain of the meningococcal microbe against which the vaccine offers protection.

This informative press release figured prominently in the mass media. This upset the owner of the pharmaceutical company who had imported the meningococcal vaccine. He tried repeatedly to see us. The secretary replied that the administration of the organization only meets with representatives of the Association of Pharmaceutical Companies about matters relating to the health sector.

Spring came and national elections were held. PASOK was again voted into power. A new Minister of Health was appointed, Alekos Papadopoulos. As soon as he took over the ministry, he asked me to draw up two proposals, one concerning the curtailment of pharmaceutical expenses, and another concerning the modernization of the National Health System. In very little time, my colleagues and I wrote up the proposals and handed them in. I was never informed whether the minster agreed or disagreed with our perspectives. They never called me in to discuss them. From the prevailing atmosphere, however, messages could be discerned that I was falling out of grace as the president of the National Organization for Medicines.

Toward the end of spring, the industrialist who had imported the vaccine for meningococcus succeeded in getting an appointment to see us. He had formed his own association of pharmaceutical companies, as he represented many companies, and he came as their representative. I received him together with the vice-president of the organization. He tried to persuade us to modify the decision of the board of directors concerning the vaccine for meningococcus, that is, he asked that we allow it to circulate freely in the marketplace and that it not be administered through health centers only when an epidemic occurs. We explicitly told him that this was not possible, because if we carried out his wishes, we would be abolishing the organization's role as the protector of public health. With quite a lot of nerve, he said to me: "If you do not grant my request, Mr. President, by the end of August your participation in the organization will be a thing of the past." Despite his reproaches, we remained steadfast in our attitude.

Indeed, at the beginning of August, 2000, while I was on vacation in Kythira, the secretary of the pathophysiology department notified me that the rector had forwarded me the final determination arrived at by the Ministry of Education, stating that I could not serve even as an unsalaried president of the National Organization for Medicines, as long as I still held the position of chairman of the Pathophysiology department. The rector had only now forwarded me the determination by the ministry that had in fact been made six months earlier, on February 20, 2000. What should one make of these events? It is obvious, even to someone with no knowledge of medicines and their regulation, that the pharmaceutical circuit wanted to keep me on hold, almost as a hostage. They had been keeping track of how cooperative I was with the pharmaceutical industry. When they saw that I held to my position, they made use of the fabrication that I was not the legal president of the National Organization for Medicines, and the ministerial determination that had been on hold was now released. I tried to get in touch with the government, with the people who had made the decision to appoint me, but everyone was away on vacation.

Since I did not want to give up my main occupation, that of physician, teacher, and researcher, without wasting any further time, I submitted my resignation from the position of president of the National Organization for Medicines. The only newspaper that mentioned my resignation was the far-left *Rizospastis*. The evil circuit of professors of medicine, PASOK, the opposition party and the pharmaceutical industry had triumphed. The only ones who lost, in the end, were the improperly cared for Greek patients. I have to admit that I, too, gained something. I acquired new experiences and knowledge, I tried my hand at management outside the narrow confines of medicine, and I believe I succeeded. I made new friends, and in spite of my short tenure at the National Organization for Medicines, I believe, in all modesty, that I made a small contribution to the modernization and the transparency of the organization. That experience taught me, however, how difficult the road to the modernization of our institutions is, and to what extent private interests impose themselves on the good of the public.

6.12   A Brief Foray into Politics

Every citizen, in the way he or she lives and interacts with others, embodies a set of ideological beliefs. In my professional and academic life, I always did my best and I am proud of my accomplishments as a physician, educator, and researcher. I cannot claim, however, that I was able, through my actions, teaching, and writings, to influence and improve certain practices that were not beneficial to the health system or to medical education in our country. Unfortunately, corruption, mediocrity, nepotism, and internal favoritism are still prevalent in most Greek institutions.

In 2009, close to the time of my obligatory retirement from the university, I thought it was an ideal period of my life to become actively involved in politics, in the hope that reforms that had been successfully implemented in more developed countries could be carried out effectively in Greece. Joining a political movement at that stage of my life was consistent with my belief that civilians, before entering into active politics, should first be successful in their professional lives.

In that same year, along with other professionally successful citizens, the majority of whom had not previously been involved in politics, I joined a political movement called ACTION, under the leadership of Stefanos Manos, a highly-respected and very effective politician in every ministerial post he had held. It was also novel for the political scene in Greece that the members of this movement had very different ideological backgrounds but held the same beliefs in transparency, meritocracy, hard work, and selflessness. We, the members of this movement, were progressive citizens with a deep respect for individual freedom. We wanted citizens with open eyes, not followers blinkered by party dogma. We wanted people to express themselves and to act according to their beliefs. Our priorities were the eradication of bribery, arbitrariness, and bureaucracy. We were ready to propose simple and practical ways to solve chronic, anachronistic problems and transform Greece into a contemporary European country. We supported competition and free markets operating under surveillance and regulations. We did not support closed professions. We wanted the public sector to function free of party influences, and to limit as much as possible unnecessary spending of government funds. We wanted an independent judicial system, free of influence or control by governmental or private actors.

We conveyed our beliefs and how we were planning to implement them to Greek citizens through lectures and limited television interviews. I accepted, in order to help the movement, an honorary, not electable position, on the European ballot. I visited Ioannina. I delivered lectures and gave TV interviews. Walking on the streets of my hometown, every person I met reassured me that in our prefecture we would get a significant percentage of votes. The votes our movement received were really disappointing. We failed to reach the threshold of 3% of the votes necessary for a seat in the European Parliament, garnering a country-wide total of only 38,895 votes (0.76%).

Following these results, my short-lived political career came to an abrupt end. Reconsidering why we failed, there were many reasons. We did not have strong social and economic supporters, nor did we have a well-organized network of supporters throughout the country. Our political positions frightened some people, who stood to lose certain privileges. The social media, newspapers, and TV were not friendly, nor did they promote our positions. It became apparent that amelioration of chronic problems takes time and serious effort. Furthermore, the necessity for the proposed reforms must be comprehended and believed by the majority of the population, and the politicians must be pressured to implement them.

6.13   The Hellenic National Library: Chairman
of the Board of Directors

It was late in the spring of 2011, when I got a call from the office of the Ministry of Education inviting me to have a meeting with Anna Diamantopoulos, the Minister. A couple of days later, I was in her office. She described, with the darkest of colors, the condition of the Hellenic National Library (HNL) and asked me if I was willing to take over the Chair of the board of directors of the HNL, making it clear that she would be at our side and support any action that could help overcome the obstacles and renovate the library. After giving it serious thought for several days, and despite my bitter experience as the president of the National Organization for Medicines, I accepted to serve *pro bono* as chairman. I was enthusiastic and ready to serve as a guardian of the country's intellectual property, in the historic building of the HNL. The HNL was part of a three-building complex in the center of Athens that included the National Library (NL), the central university building, and the Academy. The NL building was funded by a donation from the Vallianos Brothers, Cephalonian ship owners, and wheat merchants from the Greek Diaspora.

As soon as I took over the administration of the NL, the first problem emerged: The director of the NL services suddenly retired. According to rumors, she was tired and afraid that the new administration would require too much hard work from her. Without losing any time, we interviewed the NL staff in order to identify the most qualified employee for the position of associate general director. Only one of the public servants we interviewed was multilingual, a Ph.D. candidate in library science, and a member of the board of directors of the International Libraries Association. However, she did not have seniority in the NL hierarchy. Despite this, she was soon given the appointment, following our proposal to the Ministry of Education. Two of the senior employees, with minimal basic qualifications, filed a lawsuit at the Administrative Court. We hoped that their lawsuit would not be approved by the court and that we could continue working with the administrator we had selected.

During a subsequent visit to the library's premises, I realized that the west wing had been severely damaged by the most recent earthquake in Athens. The basement was serving as a storage area, where valuable old furniture, paintings, statues, and other objects were accumulated. In the main reading hall, the majority of the computers were of obsolete technology, and most of them malfunctioning. The whole library had only one photocopy machine which, due to lack of finances, was out of order. The administrative authorities were simply not able to buy ink and paper. Furthermore, the NL's debts were huge and the whole country was under strict European economic surveillance due to high public debt. All the odds were against us. It was obvious that we had to find methods to overcome these difficulties and fulfill some of our goals.

We immediately began negotiations with companies supplying electricity, water, telephone, and cleaning services. Our negotiations, with different providers, were fruitful and lead to the reduction of the library's annual costs by 25−30%.

Then we solicited contributions from our benefactors. With their generous help, we managed to acquire computers and photocopying machines. A painter and a sculptor, both NL employees, drew up a catalog of the library's paintings and sculptures. The owner of a moving company, a friend of mine, transported all the valuable old pieces of furniture and antiques, free of charge, from there to a building in Votanikos, part of which was bought by the previous administration with a loan from the National Bank of Greece under rather expensive terms. One and a half floors and the basement in this building were allocated to the NL.

The services for cataloging books (ISBN), periodicals (ISSN), and musical publications (ISMN) were transferred to half of the first floor. The valuable old furniture and artwork were put in the other half of the first floor, and a meeting room was created. On the ground floor, equipment for bookbinding and the conservation of old books and manuscripts was available, but unfortunately not in use. The specialists who performed this work, using many excuses, refused to move and work in this building. The rest of the first floor was a storage area, filled with boxes, papers, piles of bricks, and pieces of wood. This refuse was cleaned out with the help of the moving company. Newspapers and periodicals had been moved to the basement and were available for the public to look up information published decades earlier.

With the library's budget we were not able to service even the accumulated interest of the loan. This was another hot potato in our hands. Accompanied by the vice-chairman of the library's board, I met with the chairman of the National Bank of Greece. We explained the grave economic situation of the NL and asked him to extend the time period for the repayment of the capital and the interest of the loan. While his initial reaction was rather promising, shortly thereafter we got a negative answer to our request. The debts to the National Bank were accumulating, and the future of this real estate was not looking bright. Whether or not this real estate still belongs to the NL, or to the National Bank of Greece today is something I do not know.

At this point, it should be mentioned that this property was acquired at a time when the Ministry of Education and the previous NL administration were negotiating with the Stavros Niarchos Foundation concerning the creation of a cultural center, which was planned to host the NL and the National Opera. What caused the former administration to acquire that expensive piece of property in Votanikos is beyond my understanding. To be sure there are many explanations.

Thanks to additional benefactors we were able to accomplish the following:

- Clean the indoor and outdoor areas of the library.
- Clean and enrich the library's garden with trees, flowers, and benches, enabling outdoor reading, when the weather permitted it.
- Clean the glass roof of the library's main hall and the surrounding library marbles.
- Hire security guards for the weekends.
- Install Wi-Fi Internet connection in the main library's hall and in the garden.
- Connect all the library telephones through a telephone center.
- Create a new modern and easy-to-use website.
- Obtain a car to serve the library's transport needs.

Photo 6.3 Author at a seminar entitled "Poetry and economic crisis" handing out diplomas of appreciation to poets Nanos Valaoritis (seated) and Titos Patrikios (standing)

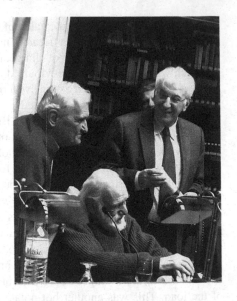

I think that our major contributions during our short time as the administration of the NL were the following: (a) we opened the library to the public by organizing cultural, academic (Photo 6.3), and scientific events, as well as regular guided tours, (b) we implemented educational programs for children and poor citizens and donated surplus literature and educational books to school libraries, (c) we promoted the services of the NL through television programs and electronic media, (d) we signed memoranda of cooperation with European and national libraries and other cultural bodies, and (e) we participated in international book fairs where we exhibited invaluable old Greek publications representing our country.

We were not able, however, to achieve our major goal: The digitization of the library's intellectual property. This project was started by the previous administration. The European funds allocated for this project accomplished the digitization of only a small portion of the library's holdings.

An architectural, static, and electric-mechanical study, concerning the restoration of the library's west wing following the damage caused by the earthquake, was performed free of charge by an architectural office. The cost of its implementation was estimated not to exceed 5 million euros. The library, through this restoration, would acquire another auditorium and plenty of additional office space, laboratories, and small meeting rooms. The Minister of Education suggested that she had this amount of money available for the realization of the project. She proposed a reputable building company that restored historic buildings to perform this work. I must admit that we were hesitant to give such an expensive project to a private company without an open and transparent competition process. This decision, seen in hindsight, was wrong. It left the historic NL's building crumbling. Then we took a second, not politically correct, step. We approached the administrators of the Stavros Niarchos Foundation and tried to convince them that it was more advantageous for the public, as well as for the foundation itself, to restore the demolished west wing of the historic library's building at a relatively low cost, rather than spend a huge sum of money to create a cultural center in an area with poor public transportation. In support of our argument, we pointed out to them how the National Library of France was restored, wing by wing, and continued functioning in the center of Paris. In addition, we emphasized that nowadays, the treasures of national libraries are digitized and immense buildings are not necessary. Unfortunately, our arguments fell on deaf ears.

It was obvious that the Stavros Niarchos Foundation had decided to move all of the NL Intellectual Property to the Stavros Niarchos Foundation Cultural Center. In the summer of 2012, the government changed. Ms. Diamantopoulos left the Ministry of Education. The new administration of the Ministry of Education was on the side of the powerful. Six months later, the new minister of education requested our resignation, without a word of gratitude. The guardians of the national intellectual treasure were defeated. And one of the three historic buildings in the center of Athens has now been abandoned to bats, rats and spiders.

To the best of my knowledge, there are no plans for the restoration of the Vallianos building or for its future function. Let us hope that a benefactor will restore it and that soon it will operate either as a library of the university or of the Academy of Athens.

6.14 Eighteen-Year Directorship of the Department of Pathophysiology: A Review

Time goes by quickly. It was 2011, the year of my retirement. It seemed like yesterday when, in 1993, I assumed responsibility for the Pathophysiology department at the Athens University Medical School. We took over an almost lifeless place, and we transformed it into a vibrant clinical service and a contemporary research environment. The patients' wards now hosted individuals with autoimmune rheumatic diseases from every corner of Greece. Biologists and young physicians worked endless hours to complete experiments toward their Ph.D. theses. The research laboratory was buzzing with life.

The team of young colleagues who came with me to Athens from the University of Ioannina, after years of difficult clinical and research work, are now senior faculty members (Photo 6.4). Their research accomplishments made them well known in the international academic community. Five years later, from the time we undertook the administration of the department of Pathophysiology, Dr. Michael (Mike) Voulgarelis, a hematologist, joined our Faculty as an Assistant Professor. He was trained in the department of Internal Medicine at the Ioannina University Medical School. He was an exceptionally efficient resident. Subsequently, he was trained in hematology in Laïko University General Hospital of Athens, a hospital known for its contributions on the molecular basis of hemoglobinopathies. As a specialist, Dr. Voulgarelis worked initially as an attending physician, under the directorship of Professor

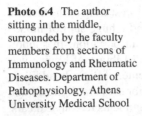

Photo 6.4 The author sitting in the middle, surrounded by the faculty members from sections of Immunology and Rheumatic Diseases. Department of Pathophysiology, Athens University Medical School

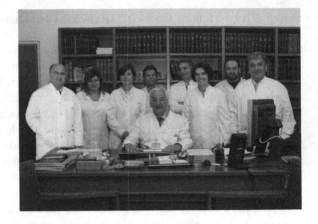

Skopouli in the department of Medicine at Evgenidio University Hospital of Athens. In the department of Pathophysiology his clinical, didactic, and research contributions in the myelodysplastic syndromes and lymphoma development in autoimmune rheumatic diseases were exemplary.

In the meantime, a new generation of clinicians and scientists is being trained and will join them in continuing to provide evidence-based clinical care to patients and in producing new scientific knowledge through research. All of them, I am sure, will keep on working, and I hope that they will continue to enhance the reputation of our department.

Some of our trainees and subsequently our collaborators became renowned senior faculty members in other Greek (Andreas Andonopoulos, Foteini N. Skopouli, George Dalekos, Maria Tektonidou and Clio Mavragani), European (Peter Katsikis, Antigoni Triantofilopoulou), and American medical institutions (Nikos Tapinos, Ioannis Dimitriou, Constantinos Petrovas, Pinelopi Kapitsinou and Issa Dahabre). Many young physicians and biologists, after doing significant research work and acquiring their Ph.D.s, decided to continue their training in the U.S. or at European centers. Today, most of them have joined the faculties of medical schools and are working at research institutes, or in the pharmaceutical industry. I'm sure that these colleagues will excuse me not to mention each one by his/her name.

Our department also had the honor of being chosen as a preferred center for rotation of medical students from the U.S., the European continent, and the U.K. Moreover, our department functioned as a center for super-specialization in autoimmune rheumatic diseases for rheumatologists working in hospitals of the National Health System. Furthermore, during this period of time, we organized many meetings, such as the VII Mediterranean Congress of Rheumatology (1994), the XVIII European Workshop for Rheumatology Research (1998), the V European Conference on Systemic Lupus Erythematosus (2002), a Symposium on Systemic Autoimmune Rheumatic Diseases (2010), and the XI International Symposium on Sjögren's Syndrome (2011).

During my tenure at the Athens University Medical School I had the honor, through invitations, to present our scientific work at different universities and research institutes in our country, as well as at universities or scientific meetings in European countries, in many states in the U.S., and in Israel, Jordan, Mexico, Argentina, Brazil, Chile, Japan, and China. Following my proposals, the University of Athens also awarded *honoris causa* doctoral degrees to Greek immunologists and internists from the Diaspora as well as to my former American teachers and collaborators.

Did I make any mistakes during my tenure? Of course I did. But none of my actions, right or wrong, were ever motivated by personal gain or self-interest. I must admit that I didn't foresee the evolution of several of my junior faculty members, whom I zealously supported, believing that they were capable of accomplishing significant academic and scientific progress. I was hoping that their promotion would give them a boost and that their performance would improve. But alas! Instead of improving, they became the black sheep of the department. Then, there was a time when I had to choose, after careful examination, two specialists, for the position of senior faculty members. Both initially collaborated effectively as teachers, clinicians, and researchers. However, as soon as they were promoted to the level of professor, one resigned from our school and emigrated to the U.S., and the other chose to move to a less demanding department of medicine in our school. The most serious mistake we continued to make during our tenure in the Athens University Medical School was not curtailing my obsessive support to candidates seeking for professorships, who were educated and worked for prolonged periods of time in famous medical centers of the West. Were we correct in selecting those candidates? I am sorry to admit that in most cases we were not. None of the selected professors from abroad developed a school of thought in his specialty. Some left the post shortly after assuming the Chair, others went into private practice, while others became the wrong prototype of a professor, due to their poor clinical skills and performance. What lesson can be drawn from these misjudgments regarding the selection of professors? Senior academics working for prolonged periods of time in demanding medical environments, when repatriated, are burned out and do not have the desire, or the strength to overcome the inevitable obstacles and difficulties they encounter in order to modernize the department for which they were selected.

These were minor mishaps, for the most part, and when all is said and done, I believe that the pluses during my years at the University of Athens far outweigh the minuses. My students, however, are the ones who will ultimately judge my eighteen-year tenure at the university as a clinician, a teacher, and a researcher.

6.15 Collecting Art: A Passion Beyond Medicine and Public Service

Medical and public service were not my only passions in life. One major passion was my love for paintings. This passion was awakened during my visits to different art galleries around the world with my mentor Normal Talal, after our scientific obligations were over. The works of some artists were most exciting to me. They spoke to me. My true love for paintings has just begun. This passion was further intensified through my association with Fotini. Her home and later ours were decorated with watercolors, oil paintings, and drawings by her mother's brother, Christos Danglis, and her cousin Stavros Baltoyiannis. Our education and ability to appreciate artwork was further enhanced by visits to exhibitions of paintings in art galleries, and by following art auctions. When, about thirty years ago, our economic situation allowed us to acquire artwork, we began to collect paintings. Our collection of paintings does not represent a special artistic period or movement. It is the result of the attraction and communication between us and what we saw portrayed on canvas. We didn't acquire paintings as a way to invest our money. Neither of us is skilled in the art of investment. Fotini had a skilled eye when it came to selecting a good piece of art, however, and whenever I was reluctant to buy a piece of art because of its price, she always encouraged me to buy it anyway. We now host in our houses hundreds of paintings by Greek and foreign artists. I will not tire the reader with the details of how we acquired the bulk of our paintings, but will simply mention three visits to art galleries abroad that led us to acquire works of well-known, local painters—visits that remain quite vivid in my memory. One was to Rio de Janeiro, in Brazil. Fotini and I were wandering around in a safe neighborhood with nice shops, restaurants, and cafés, when we spotted an art gallery with work by naïve artists. Without a second thought we went in to see the exhibition. We were immediately attracted, and our gaze was transfixed by a painting by Gerson Alves de Souza, an expressionist. The price was relatively high for our purse strings. I proposed to the owner of the gallery that I buy the painting for half of the asking price. I left the gallery after giving him all my contact details. In the evening the painting was ours. Our second fond encounter with a painting was with a famous Hungarian artist in Budapest. After I delivered the lecture I had been invited to give, Fotini and I were exploring the attractive neighborhood of Buda. In the shop-window of a gallery, we spotted a painting that drew our interest. We went into the gallery, and we found out that it was a painting by Mixaly Schener, one of the most important Hungarian expressionist painters, who was also a sculptor. His work is characterized by traditional themes in combination with rich fantasy. The price of that particular painting was relatively low, and without bargaining we acquired that beautiful piece of art. A third favorite painting of ours was acquired at a gallery in Boston. This painting was the work of Todd Mackie, a well-known artist at that time who, by the use of a small number of elements or "keys," keeps hidden a lot more than you can see at first glance. We are proud that our collection hosts important paintings. The artwork was all done in the twentieth century. In addition, our collection hosts artwork donated to us by certain artists. The major donor of her artwork to us was Véronique Youinnou, the wife of Pierre Youinnou, the professor of immunology whose laboratory I worked at as professeur associé for a year in Brest. Our art collection is on exhibit in our homes in Athens and in Ioannina, and some of the paintings adorn Niki's home in Bethesda.

To be surrounded by artwork gives us great pleasure and brightens our mood. This, however, is a rather narrow point of view when it comes to an art collection. Thinking about the future of our collection, we attempted to develop a non-profit foundation. In this way, we could make this collection available to the public. In our efforts to implement this goal, we consulted economist and lawyer friends. They were all discouraging our plans. They warned us that by doing this we would create a heavy burden for our children's shoulders. For the time being, the future of this collection seems uncertain.

6.16 The Academy of Athens: Reaching the "Top"

What does "reaching the top" mean for a person? For some people, it means financial enrichment, for others, a position in the Parliament or a minister's Chair, and for some others, it means joining the "immortals" of the highest academic institution in our country: The Academy of Athens. My long-time goal was to become part of the Academy. I felt I was deserving that nomination because of my contribution to patients' care, my dedication to educating medical students and young physicians, and the international recognition of my research in the field of autoimmune rheumatic disorders. This goal became my aspiration when I was nominated, in my early forties, as a corresponding member of the Academy. This distinction was given to me based solely on my personal achievements. It was an experience that generated in my heart a profound respect for the Academy of Athens, ignoring the fact that many distinguished professors of medicine had never even passed through the doors of this prominent institution.

In the late 1990s, I got a call from Professor Nikos Matsaniotis, who was secretary general of the Academy at that time. He informed me that the Chair of internal medicine at the Academy of Athens had been announced, and suggested that I should apply for the position. His words still ring clearly to my ears: "You may not be elected this time, since you are young, but your candidacy will give the possibility to the members of the Academy to notice your important contributions to medicine and particularly to the pathophysiology of autoimmune rheumatic diseases." Six candidates applied for the Chair. Two of them, both a lot older than me, had outstanding contributions to medicine; one had invented the aortic balloon for handling patients with congestive heart failure, and the other had developed the activated anthrax columns for hemodialysis of patients with renal failure. And what was the result of this election? No one was elected! I'm afraid that my candidacy played a key role. Ten years later, I got another call from Nikos Matsaniotis. This time, I didn't give him an answer over the phone. I went to his office. We had long discussions concerning the candidacy of my colleague Charis Roussos (ChR). I argued that it was the turn of ChR to apply for the Chair. I reminded Professor Matsaniotis that ChR had instituted contemporary ICUs in our country and that his students were now the heads of ICUs in almost all tertiary hospitals in Greece. I also reminded him that ChR's conscientious and steady support of my candidacy for the professorship in pathophysiology helped me move from the Ioannina University Medical School to the Athens University Medical School. For all these reasons, we decided that it would not be very ethical, on my part, to compete against ChR for the same Chair at the Academy. After two attempts, ChR was elected a life member of the Academy of Athens.

It must be said that ChR tried to convince his peers in the Academy's section of basic sciences to announce a Chair for which I could apply. Two academicians were strongly against my candidacy. The most vehement opponent of my candidacy was a powerful member of the Academy. ChR managed to soften his opposition to my candidacy by supporting his protégé to become a member of the Academy. I must confess that the whole idea of becoming an object of wheeling-and-dealing, hurt my pride. I was plagued by doubts, and began wondering if I really wanted to become a member of the Academy. To be honest, there were moments when I was on the verge of retiring from my candidacy. My fervent supporters encouraged me by insisting that I deserved to become a member of the Academy.

I followed the protocol and telephoned all the electors for an interview. Some of them told me that my accomplishments were well known and that I should therefore not waste my time and theirs for an unnecessary interview. Others interviewed me in a polite and academically proper manner. I will never forget an interview with an academician, an astrophysicist, who coolly told me: "Your academic accomplishments are superb, but I can't say the same about your ethics." To whom I immediately responded: "I have, throughout my life, religiously upheld the highest moral and ethical standards." "But please tell me," I continued, "on what facts do you base this slander?" Almost whispering, he said: "On the fact that ChR is supporting your candidacy." I got up from my chair, furious, and I told him: "Shame on you, you are badmouthing your colleague in his absence. I don't care if you vote for me or not, but I will not allow you to slander me, and if you repeat these words, we will see each other in court."

In February of 2017, I was elected to the Chair of Medical Sciences-Immunology in Science Section of the Academy of Athens. Three quarters of the electors voted for me (Photo 6.5).

At this point, I think, I should explain how the Academy of Athens functions. The permanent members, according to their specialty, belong to one of the three following sections: (A) Sciences, (B) Arts and Letters, and (C) Ethical and Political Sciences. The total number of permanent members is sixty. This number is seldom reached. The members of the sections meet once or twice a month according to the quantity of issues they have to discuss. They confer awards for distinguished research papers, or other publications, or works. They also award individuals, or institutions for major achievements, propose the establishment of new Chairs and prioritize, according to their achievements, candidates for an announced Chair. In addition, they nominate individuals from the international scientific community to become corresponding members, foreign fellows, or honorary members, according to the significance of their professional and/or scientific contributions. All decisions in all sections are approved or rejected by the general assembly of all the permanent members of the Academy.

Photo 6.5   Author lecturing
in the Academy of Athens

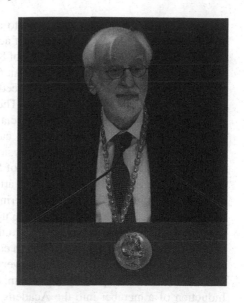

Has my experience been pleasant, fruitful, or educational during the years I've been a member of the Academy? I'm afraid not. Shouting, arguments, and angry statements make the sessions of the section and the general assembly unpleasant and very tiresome. The major problem of the Academy is that the candidates with the best scientific and/or professional records are not always elected. One important factor is the degree of genuine and consistent support a candidate receives from members of the Academy in a scientifically related field. Unfortunately, there is a major impact affecting the election procedure caused by the support of external political or religious influences for a candidate regardless of his/her accomplishments. One might ask why academicians succumb to these pressures. Quite probably because they, themselves, were elected through the intervention of extra-institutional forces. Thus, during their tenure at the Academy, they remain subservient to these forces. Still other members do the bidding of powerful individuals because they expect something in return. Also worth noting is the fact that some academicians simply vote for their friends, hoping that their power in the Academy will be increased. Because of these circumstances, internationally renowned scientists with innovative published work are not elected to the Academy, and therefore, the reputation of the highest educational institution in Greece is seriously damaged.

In light of all this, an issue raises: What makes one remain an active member in the Academy? In my case, the answer is that I hope that a different voice can be heard. I also don't want to give anyone the satisfaction of getting rid of me. Furthermore, it gives me pleasure to be able to freely express my opinions, without expecting personal gain or having ulterior motives. "Do you think you could really turn things around?", a friend asked me. That is not an easy task. Many things need to change. Every change will be fought by opponents. Nevertheless, let me mention just a few.

The Academy functions according to a law that was passed in the late 1920s. This law should be updated. The idea of active membership for life should be abandoned. Academicians reaching the age of 80 years old should automatically become inactive members. Candidates older than 60 years of age should not be allowed to apply for membership. All decisions need to be taken with transparency and with an open and adequately justified vote. The three existing sections of the Academy should be increased. For example, physicians, dentists, pharmacists, and other health professionals could constitute a section called the National Academy of Medicine. Biologists, biochemists, geneticists, physicists, chemists, and mathematicians could then constitute the National Academy of Science, while engineers and other technology experts, computer scientists, and artists could be grouped together in a section called the National Academy of Engineering and the Arts. Historians, archaeologists, linguists, poets, and writers could make up another section, the National Academy of Letters, while lawyers, economists, ethicists, sociologists, and political scientists could constitute yet another section called the National Academy of Ethics and Political Sciences. The decisions of every single section of the Academy should be respected and accepted by the administration, except if a decision is unlawful. Induction of a member into the Academy should simply be the highest academic award, without any financial compensation. These and other changes will modernize the Academy, and its reputation will then reach the highest level it deserves. Do I think that these changes will be realized? No, I do not, at least not easily. Why? Because the majority of the members are over 75 years old, very close to the age I am proposing for retirement. Others, perhaps some potential candidates, will oppose to these changes because, despite the fact that they are over 80 years old, they hope to be elected members of the Academy. And some others will be against these reforms because they don't want to lose their handsome tax-free monthly compensation.

Summing up the long journey of my life which was a hurdle race of many "kilometers" of hard work and absolute devotion, I finally reached the top. But even at the top, there is still work to be done. And I will continue, as always, my pursuit of excellence.

Printed in the United States
by Baker & Taylor Publisher Services